CONTENTS

INTRODUCTION

The Gourmia air fryer is an easy way to cook delicious healthy meals. Rather than cooking the food in oil and hot fat that may affect your health, the machine uses rapid hot air to circulate around and cook meals. This allows the outside of your food to be crispy and also makes sure that the inside layers are cooked through.

Gourmia air fryer allows us to cook almost everything and a lot of dishes. We can use the Gourmia air fryer to cook Meat, vegetables, poultry, fruit, fish and a wide variety of desserts. It is possible to prepare your entire meals, starting from appetizers to main courses as well as desserts. Not to mention, Gourmia air fryer also allows home made preserves or even delicious sweets and cakes.

How Does Gourmia air fryer Works?

The technology of the Gourmia air fryer is very simple. Fried foods get their crunchy texture because hot oil heats foods quickly and evenly on their surface. Oil is an excellent heat conductor, which helps with fast and simultaneous cooking across all of the ingredients. For decades cooks have used convection ovens to try to mimic the effects of frying or cooking the whole surface of the food. But the air never circulates quickly enough to achieve that delicious surface crisp we all love in fried foods.

With this mechanism, the air is circulated on high degrees, up to 200° C, to "air fry" any food such as fish, chicken or chips, etc. This technology has changed the whole idea of cooking by reducing the fat up to 80% compared to old-fashioned deep fat frying.

The Gourmia air fryer cooking releases the heat through a heating element which cooks the food in a healthier and more appropriate way. There's also an exhaust fan right above the cooking chamber which provides the food required airflow. This way food is cooked with constant heated air. This leads to the same heating temperature reaching every single part of the food that is being cooked. So, this is only grill and the exhaust fan that is helping the Gourmia air fryer to boost air at a constantly high speed in order to cook healthy food with less fat.

The internal pressure increases the temperature that will then be controlled by the exhaust system. Exhaust fan also releases filtered extra air to cook the food in a much healthier way. Gourmia air fryer has no odor at all and it is absolutely harmless making it user and environment-friendly.

Benefits of the Gourmia air fryer
- Healthier, oil-free meals
- It eliminates cooking odors through internal air filters
- Makes cleaning easier due to lack of oil grease
- Air Fryers are able to bake, grill, roast and fry providing more options
- A safer method of cooking compared to deep frying with exposed hot oil
- Has the ability to set and leave as most models and it includes a digital timer

The Gourmia air fryer is an all-in-one that allows cooking to be easy and quick. It also leads to a lot of possibilities once you get to know it. Once you learn the basics and become familiar with your Gourmia air fryer, you can feel free to experiment and modify the recipes in the way you prefer. You can prepare a wide number of dishes in the Gourmia air fryer and you can adapt your favorite stove-top dish so it becomes air fryer–friendly. It all boils down to variety and lots of options, right?

Cooking perfect and delicious as well as healthy meals has never been easier. You can see how this recipe collection proves itself.

Enjoy!

BREAKFAST & BRUNCH RECIPES

1. Tofu And Mushroom Omelet

Servings:2
Cooking Time:28 Minutes
Ingredients:
- ¼ of onion, chopped
- 8 ounces silken tofu, pressed and sliced
- 3½ ounces fresh mushrooms, sliced
- 3 eggs, beaten
- 2 tablespoons milk
- 2 teaspoons canola oil
- 1 garlic clove, minced
- Salt and black pepper, to taste

Directions:
1. Preheat the Air fryer to 360 °F and grease an Air Fryer pan.
2. Heat oil in the Air Fryer pan and add garlic and onion.
3. Cook for about 3 minutes and stir in the tofu and mushrooms.
4. Season with salt and black pepper and top with the beaten eggs.
5. Cook for about 25 minutes, poking the eggs twice in between.
6. Dish out and serve warm.

2. Cheddar & Bacon Quiche

Servings: 4
Cooking Time: 30 Minutes
Ingredients:
- 3 tbsp. Greek yogurt
- ½ cup grated cheddar cheese
- 3 oz. chopped bacon
- 4 eggs, beaten
- ¼ tsp. garlic powder
- Pinch of black pepper
- 1 shortcrust pastry
- ¼ tsp. onion powder
- ¼ tsp. sea salt
- Some flour for sprinkling

Directions:
1. Pre-heat your Air Fryer at 330°F.
2. Take 8 ramekins and grease with a little oil. Coat with a sprinkling of flour, tapping to remove any excess.
3. Cut the short crust pastry in 8 and place each piece at the bottom of each ramekin.
4. Put all of the other ingredients in a bowl and combine well. Spoon equal amounts of the filling into each piece of pastry.
5. Cook the ramekins in the Air Fryer for 20 minutes.

3. Cheesy Sandwich

Servings: 1
Cooking Time:18 Minutes
Ingredients:
- 2 bread slices
- 2 cheddar cheese slices
- 2 tsp. butter
- A pinch of sweet paprika

Directions:
1. Spread butter on bread slices, add cheddar cheese on one, sprinkle paprika, top with the other bread slices, cut into 2 halves; arrange them in your air fryer and cook at 370 °F, for 8 minutes; flipping them once, arrange on a plate and serve.

4. Cristy's Pancakes

Servings: 1
Cooking Time: 10 Minutes
Ingredients:
- 1 scoop of genX Vanilla
- 1 tbsp or hazelnut meal
- 2 tbsp water
- 1 egg

Directions:

1. Add the ingredients together in a bowl and mix together.
2. Pour the mixture into a frying pan, cook on a medium heat for approximately 2 to 3 minutes on each side. (Watch carefully as it may burn quickly.)
3. Serve buttered with a handful of mixed berries.

5. Mascarpone Bites

Servings: 4
Cooking Time: 3 Minutes
Ingredients:
- 4 tablespoons cream cheese
- 4 teaspoons Erythritol
- ¼ teaspoon vanilla extract
- 1 tablespoon mascarpone
- 4 tablespoons coconut milk
- 4 tablespoons almond flour

Directions:
1. Mix up cream cheese with Erythritol, vanilla extract, and mascarpone. Make the cheesecake balls (bites) and put them on the baking paper. Refrigerate the cheesecake balls for 10-15 minutes. Then preheat the air fryer to 300F. Dip the frozen bites in the coconut milk and coat in the almond flour. Cook them in the air fryer for 3 minutes.

6. Avocado And Cabbage Salad

Servings: 4
Cooking Time: 15 Minutes
Ingredients:
- 2 cups red cabbage, shredded
- A drizzle of olive oil
- 1 red bell pepper, sliced
- 1 small avocado, peeled, pitted and sliced
- Salt and black pepper to the taste

Directions:
1. Grease your air fryer with the oil, add all the ingredients, toss, cover and cook at 400 degrees F for 15 minutes. Divide into bowls and serve cold for breakfast.

7. Potato Rosti

Servings:2
Cooking Time: 15 Minutes
Ingredients:
- 1 teaspoon olive oil
- ½ pound russet potatoes, peeled and roughly grated
- 1 tablespoon fresh chives, finely chopped
- Salt and ground black pepper, as required
- 2 tablespoons sour cream
- 3½ ounces smoked salmon, cut into slices

Directions:
1. Set the temperature of Air Fryer to 355 degrees F. Grease a pizza pan with the olive oil.
2. In a large bowl, mix together the potatoes, chives, salt, and black pepper.
3. Place the potato mixture into the prepared pizza pan.
4. Arrange the pan in an Air Fryer basket.
5. Air Fry for about 15 minutes or until the top becomes golden brown.
6. Cut the potato rosti into wedges.
7. Top with the sour cream and smoked salmon slices and serve immediately.

8. Cheese Stuff Peppers

Servings: 8
Cooking Time: 8 Minutes
Ingredients:

- 8 small bell pepper, cut the top of peppers
- 3.5 oz feta cheese, cubed
- 1 tbsp olive oil
- 1 tsp Italian seasoning
- 1 tbsp parsley, chopped
- ¼ tsp garlic powder
- Pepper
- Salt

Directions:

1. In a bowl, toss cheese with oil and seasoning.
2. Stuff cheese in each bell peppers and place into the air fryer basket.
3. Cook at 400 F for 8 minutes.
4. Serve and enjoy.

9. Parmesan Muffins

Servings: 4
Cooking Time: 15 Minutes
Ingredients:

- 2 eggs, whisked
- Cooking spray
- 1 and ½ cups coconut milk
- 1 tablespoon baking powder
- 4 ounces baby spinach, chopped
- 2 ounces parmesan cheese, grated
- 3 ounces almond flour

Directions:

1. In a bowl, mix all the ingredients except the cooking spray and whisk really well. Grease a muffin pan that fits your air fryer with the cooking spray, divide the muffins mix, introduce the pan in the air fryer, cook at 380 degrees F for 15 minutes, divide between plates and serve.

10. Cheddar Tomatoes Hash

Servings: 4
Cooking Time: 25 Minutes
Ingredients:

- 2 tablespoons olive oil
- 1 pound tomatoes, chopped
- ½ pound cheddar, shredded
- 2 tablespoons chives, chopped
- Salt and black pepper to the taste
- 6 eggs, whisked

Directions:

1. Add the oil to your air fryer, heat it up at 350 degrees F, add the tomatoes, eggs, salt and pepper and whisk. Also add the cheese on top and sprinkle the chives on top. Cook for 25 minutes, divide between plates and serve for breakfast.

11. Blueberry Cream Cheese With French Toast

Servings:4
Cooking Time: 15 Minutes
Ingredients:

- 4 slices bread
- 3 tbsp sugar
- 1½ cups corn flakes
- ⅓ cup milk
- ¼ tsp nutmeg
- 4 tbsp berry-flavored cheese
- ¼ tsp salt

Directions:

1. Preheat your air fryer to 400 F. In a bowl, mix sugar, eggs, nutmeg, salt and milk. In a separate bowl, mix blueberries and cheese. Take 2 bread slices and pour the blueberry mixture over the slices.
2. Top with the milk mixture. Cover with the remaining two slices to make sandwiches. Dredge the sandwiches over cornflakes to coat thoroughly. Lay the sandwiches in your air fryer's cooking basket and cook for 8 minutes. Serve with berries and syrup.

12. Endives Frittata

Servings: 6
Cooking Time: 15 Minutes
Ingredients:
- 1 endive, shredded
- 6 eggs, whisked
- A pinch of salt and black pepper
- 1 teaspoon sweet paprika
- 2 teaspoons cilantro, chopped
- Cooking spray

Directions:
1. In a bowl, mix all the ingredients except the cooking spray and stir well. Grease a baking pan with the cooking spray, pour the frittata mix and spread well. Put the pan in the Air Fryer and cook at 370 degrees F for 15 minutes. Divide between plates and serve them for breakfast.

13. Bacon & Eggs

Servings: 1
Cooking Time: 5 Minutes
Ingredients:
- Parsley
- Cherry tomatoes
- 1/3 oz/150g bacon
- eggs

Directions:
1. Fry up the bacon and put it to the side.
2. Scramble the eggs in the bacon grease, with some pepper and salt. If you want, scramble in some cherry tomatoes. Sprinkle with some parsley and enjoy.

14. Breakfast Muffins With Walnuts

Servings:4
Cooking Time: 15 Minutes
Ingredients:
- ¼ cup mashed banana
- ¼ cup powdered sugar
- 1 tsp milk
- 1 tsp chopped walnuts
- ½ tsp baking powder
- ¼ cup oats
- ¼ cup butter, room temperature

Directions:
1. Preheat the air fryer to 320 F. Place the sugar, walnuts, banana, and butter in a bowl and mix to combine. In another bowl, combine the flour, baking powder and oats. Combine the two mixtures and stir in milk. Pour the batter in a greased tin. Cook for 10 minutes.

15. Spinach Spread

Servings: 4
Cooking Time: 10 Minutes
Ingredients:
- 2 tablespoons coconut cream
- 3 cups spinach leaves
- 2 tablespoons cilantro
- 2 tablespoons bacon, cooked and crumbled
- Salt and black pepper to the taste

Directions:
1. In a pan that fits the air fryer, combine all the ingredients except the bacon, put the pan in the machine and cook at 360 degrees F for 10 minutes. Transfer to a blender, pulse well, divide into bowls and serve with bacon sprinkled on top.

16. Bacon Grilled Cheese

Servings:2
Cooking Time:7 Minutes
Ingredients:
- 4 slices of bread
- 1 tablespoon butter, softened
- 2 slices mild cheddar cheese
- 6 slices bacon, cooked

- 2 slices mozzarella cheese
- 1 tablespoon olive oil

Directions:
1. Preheat the Air fryer to 370 °F and grease an Air fryer basket with olive oil.
2. Spread butter onto one side of each bread slice and place in the Air Fryer basket.
3. Layer with cheddar cheese slice, followed by bacon, mozzarella cheese and close with the other bread slice.
4. Place in the Air fryer and cook for about 4 minutes.
5. Flip the sandwich and cook for 3 more minutes.
6. Remove from the Air fryer and serve.

17. Cheesy Sausage Sticks

Servings: 3
Cooking Time: 8 Minutes
Ingredients:
- 6 small pork sausages
- ½ cup almond flour
- ½ cup Mozzarella cheese, shredded
- 2 eggs, beaten
- 1 tablespoon mascarpone
- Cooking spray

Directions:
1. Pierce the hot dogs with wooden coffee sticks to get the sausages on the sticks". Then in the bowl mix up almond flour, Mozzarella cheese, and mascarpone. Microwave the mixture for 15 seconds or until you get a melted mixture. Then stir the egg in the cheese mixture and whisk it until smooth. Coat every sausage stick in the cheese mixture. Then preheat the air fryer to 375F. Spray the air fryer basket with cooking spray. Place the sausage stock in the air fryer and

cook them for 4 minutes from each side or until they are light brown.

18. Mozzarella Bell Peppers Mix

Servings: 4
Cooking Time: 15 Minutes
Ingredients:
- 1 red bell pepper, roughly chopped
- 1 celery stalk, chopped
- 2 green onions, sliced
- 2 tablespoons butter, melted
- ½ cup mozzarella cheese, shredded
- A pinch of salt and black pepper
- 6 eggs, whisked

Directions:
1. In a bowl, mix all the ingredients except the butter and whisk well. Preheat the air fryer at 360 degrees F, add the butter, heat it up, add the celery and bell peppers mix, and cook for 15 minutes, shaking the fryer once. Divide the mix between plates and serve for breakfast.

19. Tasty Egg Yolks With Squid

Servings:4
Cooking Time:20 Minutes
Ingredients:
- ½ cup self-rising flour
- 14-ounce flower squid, cleaned and dried
- 2 green chilies, seeded and chopped
- 4 raw salted egg yolks
- 2 tablespoons evaporated milk
- ½ cup chicken broth
- 1 tablespoon sugar
- 3 tablespoons olive oil
- 1 tablespoon curry powder
- Salt and black pepper, to taste

Directions:
1. Preheat the Air fryer to 355 °F and grease an Air fryer pan.

2. Place the flour in a shallow dish and keep aside.
3. Sprinkle the flower squid with salt and black pepper and coat with flour.
4. Transfer the flower squid into the Air fryer pan and cook for about 9 minutes.
5. Remove from Air fryer and keep aside
6. Heat olive oil on medium heat in a skillet and add chilies and curry leaves.
7. Cook for about 3 minutes and add egg yolks
8. Cook, stirring for about1 minute and add the chicken broth.
9. Cook for about 5 minutes, stirring continuously and add evaporated milk and sugar.
10. Mix till well combined and toss in the fried flower squid until evenly coated.
11. 1Serve immediately.

20. Okra Hash

Servings: 4
Cooking Time: 20 Minutes
Ingredients:
- 2 cups okra
- 1 tablespoon butter, melted
- 4 eggs, whisked
- A pinch of salt and black pepper

Directions:
1. Grease a pan that fits the air fryer with the butter. In a bowl, combine the okra with eggs, salt and pepper, whisk and pour into the pan. Introduce the pan in the air fryer and cook at 350 degrees F for 20 minutes. Divide the mix between plates and serve.

21. Cheese & Chicken Sandwich

Servings: 1

Cooking Time: 15 Minutes
Ingredients:
- ⅓ cup chicken, cooked and shredded
- 2 mozzarella slices
- 1 hamburger bun
- ¼ cup cabbage, shredded
- 1 tsp. mayonnaise
- 2 tsp. butter
- 1 tsp. olive oil
- ½ tsp. balsamic vinegar
- 1/4 tsp. smoked paprika
- ¼ tsp. black pepper
- ¼ tsp. garlic powder
- Pinch of salt

Directions:
1. Pre-heat your Air Fryer at 370°F.
2. Apply some butter to the outside of the hamburger bun with a brush.
3. In a bowl, coat the chicken with the garlic powder, salt, pepper, and paprika.
4. In a separate bowl, stir together the mayonnaise, olive oil, cabbage, and balsamic vinegar to make coleslaw.
5. Slice the bun in two. Start building the sandwich, starting with the chicken, followed by the mozzarella, the coleslaw, and finally the top bun.
6. Transfer the sandwich to the fryer and cook for 5 – 7 minutes.

22. Cheese Eggs And Leeks

Servings: 2
Cooking Time: 7 Minutes
Ingredients:
- 2 leeks, chopped
- 4 eggs, whisked
- ¼ cup Cheddar cheese, shredded
- ½ cup Mozzarella cheese, shredded
- 1 teaspoon avocado oil

Directions:

1. Preheat the air fryer to 400F. Then brush the air fryer basket with avocado oil and combine the eggs with the rest of the ingredients inside. Cook for 7 minutes and serve.

23. Toasties

Servings: 2
Cooking Time: 30 Minutes
Ingredients:

- ¼ cup milk or cream
- 2 sausages, boiled
- 3 eggs
- 1 slice bread, sliced lengthwise
- 4 tbsp. cheese, grated
- Sea salt to taste
- Chopped fresh herbs and steamed broccoli [optional]

Directions:

1. Pre-heat your Air Fryer at 360°F and set the timer for 5 minutes.
2. In the meantime, scramble the eggs in a bowl and add in the milk.
3. Grease three muffin cups with a cooking spray. Divide the egg mixture in three and pour equal amounts into each cup.
4. Slice the sausages and drop them, along with the slices of bread, into the egg mixture. Add the cheese on top and a little salt as desired.
5. Transfer the cups to the Fryer and cook for 15-20 minutes, depending on how firm you would like them. When ready, remove them from the fryer and serve with fresh herbs and steam broccoli if you prefer.

24. Breakfast Tea

Servings: 1
Cooking Time: 5 Minutes
Ingredients:

- 16 oz water

- 2 tea bags
- 1 tbsp ghee
- 1 tbsp coconut oil
- ½ tsp vanilla extract

Directions:

1. Make the tea and put it to one aside.
2. In a bowl, melt the ghee.
3. Add the coconut oil and vanilla to the melted ghee.
4. Pour the tea from a cup into a Nutribullet cup.
5. Screw on the lid and blend thoroughly.

25. Taj Tofu

Servings: 4
Cooking Time: 40 Minutes
Ingredients:

- 1 block firm tofu, pressed and cut into 1-inch thick cubes
- 2 tbsp. soy sauce
- 2 tsp. sesame seeds, toasted
- 1 tsp. rice vinegar
- 1 tbsp. cornstarch

Directions:

1. Set your Air Fryer at 400°F to warm.
2. Add the tofu, soy sauce, sesame seeds and rice vinegar in a bowl together and mix well to coat the tofu cubes. Then cover the tofu in cornstarch and put it in the basket of your fryer.
3. Cook for 25 minutes, giving the basket a shake at five-minute intervals to ensure the tofu cooks evenly.

26. Garlicky Chicken On Green Bed

Servings:1
Cooking Time: 20 Minutes
Ingredients:

- ½ cup shredded romaine
- 3 large kale leaves, chopped

- 4 oz chicken breasts, cut into cubes
- 3 tbsp olive oil, divided
- 1 tsp balsamic vinegar
- 1 garlic clove, minced
- Salt and pepper, to taste

Directions:

1. Place the chicken, 1 tbsp olive oil, salt, garlic, and pepper in a bowl. Toss to combine.
2. Put on a lined baking dish and cook for 14 minutes at 390F in the air fryer. Place the greens in a bowl. Add in the remaining olive oil and balsamic vinegar. Top with the chicken.

27. Scrambled Eggs

Servings: 2
Cooking Time: 6 Minutes
Ingredients:

- 4 eggs
- 1/4 tsp garlic powder
- 1/4 tsp onion powder
- 1 tbsp parmesan cheese
- Pepper
- Salt

Directions:

1. Whisk eggs with garlic powder, onion powder, parmesan cheese, pepper, and salt.
2. Pour egg mixture into the air fryer baking dish.
3. Place dish in the air fryer and cook at 360 F for 2 minutes. Stir quickly and cook for 3-4 minutes more.
4. Stir well and serve.

28. Italian Chicken

Servings: 4
Cooking Time: 20 Minutes
Ingredients:

- 4 chicken thighs
- ¼ tsp onion powder
- ½ tsp garlic powder
- 2 ½ tsp dried Italian herbs
- 2 tbsp butter, melted

Directions:

1. Brush chicken with melted butter.
2. Mix together Italian herbs, onion powder, and garlic powder and rub over chicken.
3. Place chicken into the air fryer basket and cook at 380 F for 20 minutes.
4. Serve and enjoy.

29. Egg In A Bread Basket

Servings:2
Cooking Time:10 Minutes
Ingredients:

- 2 bread slices
- 1 bacon slice, chopped
- 4 tomato slices
- 1 tablespoon Mozzarella cheese, shredded
- 2 eggs
- ½ tablespoon olive oil
- 1/8 teaspoon maple syrup
- 1/8 teaspoon balsamic vinegar
- ¼ teaspoon fresh parsley, chopped
- Salt and black pepper, to taste
- 2 tablespoons mayonnaise

Directions:

1. Preheat the Air fryer to 320 °F and grease 2 ramekins lightly.
2. Place 1 bread slice in each prepared ramekin and add bacon and tomato slices.
3. Top evenly with the Mozzarella cheese and crack 1 egg in each ramekin.
4. Drizzle with balsamic vinegar and maple syrup and season with parsley, salt and black pepper.
5. Arrange the ramekins in an Air fryer basket and cook for about 10 minutes.

6. Top with mayonnaise and serve immediately.

30. Carrot Oatmeal

Servings: 4
Cooking Time: 15 Minutes
Ingredients:
- 2 cups almond milk
- ½ cup steel cut oats
- 1 cup carrots, shredded
- 1 teaspoon cardamom, ground
- 2 teaspoons sugar
- Cooking spray

Directions:
1. Spray your air fryer with cooking spray, add all ingredients, toss, and cover.
2. Cook at 365 degrees F for 15 minutes.
3. Divide into bowls and serve.

31. Puffed Egg Tarts

Servings:4
Cooking Time:42 Minutes
Ingredients:
- 1 sheet frozen puff pastry half, thawed and cut into 4 squares
- ¾ cup Monterey Jack cheese, shredded and divided
- 4 large eggs
- 1 tablespoon fresh parsley, minced
- 1 tablespoon olive oil

Directions:
1. Preheat the Air fryer to 390 °F
2. Place 2 pastry squares in the air fryer basket and cook for about 10 minutes.
3. Remove Air fryer basket from the Air fryer and press each square gently with a metal tablespoon to form an indentation.
4. Place 3 tablespoons of cheese in each hole and top with 1 egg each.
5. Return Air fryer basket to Air fryer and cook for about 11 minutes.
6. Remove tarts from the Air fryer basket and sprinkle with half the parsley.
7. Repeat with remaining pastry squares, cheese and eggs.
8. Dish out and serve warm.

LUNCH & DINNER RECIPES

32. 'no Potato' Shepherd's Pie

Servings: 6
Cooking Time: 70 Minutes
Ingredients:
- 1 lb lean ground beef
- 8 oz low-carb mushroom sauce mix
- ¼ cup ketchup
- 1 lb package frozen mixed vegetables
- 1 lb Aitkin's low-carb bake mix or equivalent

Directions:
1. Preheat your fryer to 375°F/190°C.
2. Prepare the bake mix according to package Directions:. Layer into the skillet base.
3. Cut the dough into triangles and roll them from base to tip. Set to the side.
4. Brown the ground beef with the salt. Stir in the mushroom sauce, ketchup and mixed vegetables.
5. Bring the mixture to the boil and reduce the heat to medium, cover and simmer until tender.
6. Put the dough triangles on top of the mixture, tips pointing towards the center.
7. Bake for 60 minutes until piping hot and serve!

33. Beef And Tomato Mix

Servings: 4
Cooking Time: 25 Minutes
Ingredients:
- 1 and ½ pounds beef stew meat, cubed
- ½ cup green onions, chopped
- 3 tablespoons butter, melted
- ½ cup celery stalks, chopped
- 1 garlic clove, minced
- ½ teaspoon Italian seasoning

- 15 ounces keto tomato sauce
- Salt and black pepper to the taste

Directions:
1. Heat up a pan that fits your air fryer with the butter over medium heat, add the meat, toss and brown for 5 minutes. Add the rest of the ingredients, toss, introduce the pan in the fryer and cook at 390 degrees F for 20 minutes. Divide into bowls and serve for lunch.

34. Lamb Satay

Servings: 2
Cooking Time: 25 Minutes
Ingredients:
- ¼ tsp. cumin
- 1 tsp ginger
- ½ tsp. nutmeg
- Salt and pepper
- 2 boneless lamb steaks
- Olive oil cooking spray

Directions:
1. Combine the cumin, ginger, nutmeg, salt and pepper in a bowl.
2. Cube the lamb steaks and massage the spice mixture into each one.
3. Leave to marinate for ten minutes, then transfer onto metal skewers.
4. Pre-heat the fryer at 400°F.
5. Spritz the skewers with the olive oil cooking spray, then cook them in the fryer for eight minutes.
6. Take care when removing them from the fryer and serve with the low-carb sauce of your choice.

35. Spring Onions And Shrimp Mix

Servings: 4
Cooking Time: 15 Minutes
Ingredients:

- 2 cups baby spinach
- ¼ cup veggie stock
- 2 tomatoes, cubed
- 1 tablespoon garlic, minced
- 15 ounces shrimp, peeled and deveined
- 4 spring onions, chopped
- ½ teaspoon cumin, ground
- 1 tablespoon lemon juice
- 2 tablespoons cilantro, chopped
- Salt and black pepper to the taste

Directions:
1. In a pan that fits your air fryer, mix all the ingredients except the cilantro, toss, introduce in the air fryer and cook at 360 degrees F for 15 minutes. Add the cilantro, stir, divide into bowls and serve for lunch.

36. Sweet Potatoes

Servings: 4
Cooking Time: 55 Minutes
Ingredients:
- 2 potatoes, peeled and cubed
- 4 carrots, cut into chunks
- 1 head broccoli, cut into florets
- 4 zucchinis, sliced thickly
- Salt and pepper to taste
- ¼ cup olive oil
- 1 tbsp. dry onion powder

Directions:
1. Pre-heat the Air Fryer to 400°F.
2. In a baking dish small enough to fit inside the fryer, add all the ingredients and combine well.
3. Cook for 45 minutes in the fryer, ensuring the vegetables are soft and the sides have browned before serving.

37. Salmon Salad

Servings: 4

Cooking Time: 8 Minutes
Ingredients:
- 4 salmon fillets, boneless
- 2 tablespoons olive oil
- Salt and black pepper to the taste
- 3 cups kale leaves, shredded
- 2 teaspoons balsamic vinegar

Directions:
1. Put the fish in your air fryer's basket, season with salt and pepper, drizzle half of the oil over them, cook at 400 degrees F for 4 minutes on each side, cool down and cut into medium cubes. In a bowl, mix the kale with salt, pepper, vinegar, the rest of the oil and the salmon, toss gently and serve for lunch.

38. Radish And Tuna Salad

Servings: 2
Cooking Time: 8 Minutes
Ingredients:
- ½ cup radish sprouts
- 8 oz tuna, smoked, boneless and shredded
- 1 egg, beaten
- 1 tablespoon coconut flour
- ½ teaspoon ground coriander
- ½ teaspoon lemon zest, grated
- 1 tablespoon olive oil
- ½ teaspoon salt
- 1 tablespoon lemon juice
- ½ cup radish, sliced

Directions:
1. Mix up the tuna with coconut flour, ground coriander, lemon zest, and egg. Stir the mixture until homogenous. Preheat the air fryer to 400F. Then make the small tuna balls and put them in the hot air fryer. Sprinkle the tuna balls with ½ tablespoon of olive oil. Cook the tuna

balls for 8 minutes. Flip the tuna balls on another side after 4 minutes of cooking. Meanwhile, mix up together radish sprouts and radish. Sprinkle the mixture with remaining olive oil, salt, and lemon juice. Shake it well. Then top the salad with tuna balls.

39. Coconut Chicken

Servings: 4
Cooking Time: 20 Minutes
Ingredients:
- 4 chicken breasts, skinless, boneless and cubed
- Salt and black pepper to the taste
- ¼ cup coconut cream
- 1 teaspoon olive oil
- 1 and ½ teaspoon sweet paprika

Directions:
1. Grease a pan that fits your air fryer with the oil, mix all the ingredients inside, introduce the pan in the fryer and cook at 370 degrees F for 17 minutes. Divide between plates and serve for lunch.

40. Potatoes And Calamari Stew

Servings: 4
Cooking Time: 16 Minutes
Ingredients:
- 10 ounces calamari, cut into strips
- 1 cup red wine
- 1 cup water
- 2 tablespoons olive oil
- 2 teaspoons pepper sauce
- 1 tablespoon hot sauce
- 1 tablespoon sweet paprika
- 1 tablespoon tomato sauce
- Salt and black pepper to taste
- ½ bunch cilantro, chopped
- 2 garlic cloves, minced
- 1 yellow onion, chopped

- 4 potatoes, cut into quarters.

Directions:
1. Place all the ingredients in a pan that fits the air fryer and toss.
2. Put the pan in the fryer and cook at 400 degrees F for 16 minutes.
3. Divide the stew between bowls and serve.

41. Duck Fat Ribeye

Servings: 1
Cooking Time: 20 Minutes
Ingredients:
- One 16-oz ribeye steak (1 - 1 ¼ inch thick)
- 1 tbsp duck fat (or other high smoke point oil like peanut oil)
- ½ tbsp butter
- ½ tsp thyme, chopped
- Salt and pepper to taste

Directions:
1. Preheat a skillet in your fryer at 400°F/200°C.
2. Season the steaks with the oil, salt and pepper. Remove the skillet from the fryer once pre-heated.
3. Put the skillet on your stove top burner on a medium heat and drizzle in the oil.
4. Sear the steak for 1-4 minutes, depending on if you like it rare, medium or well done.
5. Turn over the steak and place in your fryer for 6 minutes.
6. Take out the steak from your fryer and place it back on the stove top on low heat.
7. Toss in the butter and thyme and cook for 3 minutes, basting as you go along.
8. Rest for 5 minutes and serve.

42. Beef Tenderloin & Peppercorn Crust

Servings: 6

Cooking Time: 45 Minutes

Ingredients:

- 2 lb. beef tenderloin
- 2 tsp. roasted garlic, minced
- 2 tbsp. salted butter, melted
- 3 tbsp. ground 4-peppercorn blender

Directions:

1. Remove any surplus fat from the beef tenderloin.
2. Combine the roasted garlic and melted butter to apply to your tenderloin with a brush.
3. On a plate, spread out the peppercorns and roll the tenderloin in them, making sure they are covering and clinging to the meat.
4. Cook the tenderloin in your fryer for twenty-five minutes at 400°F, turning halfway through cooking.
5. Let the tenderloin rest for ten minutes before slicing and serving.

43. Sage Chicken Escallops

Servings: 4

Cooking Time: 45 Minutes

Ingredients:

- 4 skinless chicken breasts
- 2 eggs, beaten
- ½ cup flour
- 6 sage leaves
- ¼ cup bread crumbs
- ¼ cup parmesan cheese
- Cooking spray

Directions:

1. Cut the chicken breasts into thin, flat slices.
2. In a bowl, combine the parmesan with the sage.
3. Add in the flour and eggs and sprinkle with salt and pepper as desired. Mix well.
4. Dip chicken in the flour-egg mixture.
5. Coat the chicken in the panko bread crumbs.
6. Spritz the inside of the Air Fryer with cooking spray and set it to 390°F, allowing it to warm.
7. Cook the chicken for 20 minutes.
8. When golden, serve with fried rice.

44. Meatballs, Tomato Sauce

Servings: 4

Cooking Time: 245 Minutes

Ingredients:

- 1 lb. lean beef; ground
- 3 green onions; chopped.
- 2 garlic cloves; minced
- 1 egg yolk
- 1/4 cup bread crumbs
- 1 tbsp. olive oil
- 16 oz. tomato sauce
- 2 tbsp. mustard
- Salt and black pepper to the taste

Directions:

1. In a bowl; mix beef with onion, garlic, egg yolk, bread crumbs, salt and pepper; stir well and shape medium meatballs out of this mix.
2. Grease meatballs with the oil, place them in your air fryer and cook them at 400 °F, for 10 minutes.
3. In a bowl; mix tomato sauce with mustard, whisk, add over meatballs; toss them and cook at 400 °F, for 5 minutes more. Divide meatballs and sauce on plates and serve for lunch.

45. Tuna Bake

Servings: 6

Cooking Time: 15 Minutes

Ingredients:

- 2 spring onions, diced
- 1 pound smoked tuna, boneless
- ¼ cup ricotta cheese
- 3 oz celery stalk, diced
- ½ teaspoon celery seeds
- 1 tablespoon cream cheese
- ¼ teaspoon salt
- ½ teaspoon ground paprika
- 2 tablespoons lemon juice
- 1 tablespoon ghee
- 4 oz Edam cheese, shredded

Directions:

1. Mix up celery seeds, cream cheese, ground paprika, lemon juice, and ricotta cheese. Then shred the tuna until it is smooth and add it in the cream cheese mixture. Add onion and stir the mass with the help of the spoon. Grease the air fryer pan with ghee and put the tuna mixture inside. Flatten its surface gently with the help of the spoon and top with Edam cheese. Preheat the air fryer to 360F. Place the pan with tuna melt in the air fryer and cook it for 15 minutes.

46. Eggplant Bowls

Servings: 4
Cooking Time: 15 Minutes
Ingredients:

- 2 cups eggplants, cubed
- 1 cup keto tomato sauce
- 1 teaspoon olive oil
- 1 cup mozzarella, shredded

Directions:

1. In a pan that fits the air fryer, combine all the ingredients except the mozzarella and toss. Sprinkle the cheese on top, introduce the pan in the machine and cook at 390 degrees

F for 15 minutes. Divide between plates and serve for lunch.

47. Rosemary Chicken Stew

Servings: 4
Cooking Time: 20 Minutes
Ingredients:

- 2 cups okra
- 2 garlic cloves, minced
- 1 pound chicken breasts, skinless, boneless and cubed
- 4 tomatoes, cubed
- 1 tablespoon olive oil
- 1 teaspoon rosemary, dried
- Salt and black pepper to the taste
- 1 tablespoon parsley, chopped

Directions:

1. Heat up a pan that fits your air fryer with the oil over medium-high heat, add the chicken, garlic, rosemary, salt and pepper, toss and brown for 5 minutes. Add the remaining ingredients, toss again, place the pan in the air fryer and cook at 380 degrees F for 15 minutes more. Divide the stew into bowls and serve for lunch.

48. Vegan Ravioli

Servings: 4
Cooking Time: 15 Minutes
Ingredients:

- ½ cup bread crumbs
- 2 tsp. nutritional yeast
- 1 tsp. dried basil
- 1 tsp. dried oregano
- 1 tsp. garlic powder
- Salt and pepper to taste
- ¼ cup aquafaba
- 8 oz. vegan ravioli
- Cooking spray

Directions:

1. Cover the Air Fryer basket with aluminum foil and coat with a light brushing of oil.
2. Pre-heat the Air Fryer to 400°F. Combine together the panko breadcrumbs, nutritional yeast, basil, oregano, and garlic powder. Sprinkle on salt and pepper to taste.
3. Put the aquafaba in a separate bowl. Dip the ravioli in the aquafaba before coating it in the panko mixture. Spritz with cooking spray and transfer to the Air Fryer.
4. Cook for 6 minutes ensuring to shake the Air Fryer basket halfway.

49. Cilantro Turkey Casserole

Servings: 4
Cooking Time: 25 Minutes
Ingredients:
- 2 tablespoons butter, melted
- 12 ounces cream cheese, soft
- 2 cups turkey breasts, skinless, boneless and cut into strips
- 1 cups zucchinis, sliced
- 2 teaspoons sweet paprika
- 6 ounces cheddar cheese, grated
- ¼ cup cilantro, chopped
- Salt and black pepper to the taste

Directions:
1. In a baking dish that fits your air fryer, mix the butter with turkey, cream cheese and all the other ingredients except the cheddar cheese. Sprinkle the cheddar on top, put the dish in your air fryer and cook at 360 degrees F for 25 minutes. Divide between plates and serve for lunch.

50. Cauliflower

Servings: 4
Cooking Time: 20 Minutes

Ingredients:
- 1 head cauliflower, cut into florets
- 1 tbsp. extra-virgin olive oil
- 2 scallions, chopped
- 5 cloves of garlic, sliced
- 1 ½ tbsp. tamari
- 1 tbsp. rice vinegar
- ½ tsp. sugar
- 1 tbsp. sriracha

Directions:
1. Pre-heat the Air Fryer to 400°F.
2. Put the cauliflower florets in the Air Fryer and drizzle some oil over them before cooking for 10 minutes.
3. Turn the cauliflower over, throw in the onions and garlic, and stir. Cook for another 10 minutes.
4. Mix together the rest of the ingredients in a bowl.
5. Remove the cooked cauliflower from the fryer and coat it in the sauce.
6. Return to the Air Fryer and allow to cook for another 5 minutes. Enjoy with a side of rice.

51. Cheese & Macaroni Balls

Servings: 2
Cooking Time: 25 Minutes
Ingredients:
- 2 cups leftover macaroni
- 1 cup cheddar cheese, shredded
- 3 large eggs
- 1 cup milk
- ½ cup flour
- 1 cup bread crumbs
- ½ tsp. salt
- ¼ tsp. black pepper

Directions:
1. In a bowl, combine the leftover macaroni and shredded cheese.
2. Pour the flour in a separate bowl. Put the bread crumbs in a third bowl.

Finally, in a fourth bowl, mix together the eggs and milk with a whisk.

3. With an ice-cream scoop, create balls from the macaroni mixture. Coat them the flour, then in the egg mixture, and lastly in the bread crumbs.
4. Pre-heat the Air Fryer to 365°F and cook the balls for about 10 minutes, giving them an occasional stir. Ensure they crisp up nicely.
5. Serve with the sauce of your choice.

52. Beef Pie

Servings: 4
Cooking Time: 6 Minutes
Ingredients:
- 2 cup cauliflower, boiled, mashed
- 2 oz celery stalk, chopped
- 1 cup ground beef
- ½ teaspoon salt
- ½ teaspoon ground turmeric
- 1 tablespoon coconut oil
- ½ teaspoon avocado oil
- 1 teaspoon dried parsley
- 1 tablespoon keto tomato sauce
- 1 garlic clove, diced

Directions:
1. Toss the coconut oil in the skillet and melt it over the medium heat. Then add celery stalk. Cook the vegetables for 5 minutes. Stir them from time to time. Meanwhile, brush the air fryer pan with avocado oil. Transfer the cooked vegetables in the pan and flatten them in the shape of the layer. Then put the ground beef in the pan. Add salt, parsley, and turmeric. Cook the ground meat for 10 minutes over the medium heat. Stir it from time to time. Add tomato sauce and stir well. After this, transfer the ground beef

over the vegetables. Then add garlic and top the pie with mashed cauliflower mash. Preheat the air fryer to 360F. Put the pan with shepherd pie in the air fryer and cook for 6 minutes or until you get the crunchy crust.

53. Pork Casserole

Servings: 6
Cooking Time: 30 Minutes
Ingredients:
- 1 teaspoon taco seasonings
- 1 teaspoon sesame oil
- 1 teaspoon salt
- 2 cups ground pork
- ½ cup keto tomato sauce
- 2 low carb tortillas
- ½ cup Cheddar cheese, shredded
- ¼ cup mozzarella cheese, shredded

Directions:
1. Chop the tortillas roughly. Brush the air fryer pan with sesame oil and place ½ part of chopped tortilla in it. In the mixing bowl mix up taco seasonings, ground pork, and salt. Place ½ part of ground pork over the tortillas and top it with mozzarella cheese. Then cover the cheese with remaining tortillas, ground pork, and Cheddar cheese. Pour the marinara sauce over the cheese and cover the casserole with foil. Secure the edges. Preheat the air fryer to 395F. Put the casserole in the air fryer and cook it for 20 minutes. Then remove the foil and cook it for 10 minutes more.

54. Asian Tofu Bites

Servings: 4
Cooking Time: 20 Minutes
Ingredients:

- 1 packaged firm tofu, cubed and pressed to remove excess water
- 1 tbsp. soy sauce
- 1 tbsp. ketchup
- 1 tbsp. maple syrup
- ½ tsp. vinegar
- 1 tsp. liquid smoke
- 1 tsp. hot sauce
- 2 tbsp. sesame seeds
- 1 tsp. garlic powder
- Salt and pepper to taste

Directions:
1. Pre-heat the Air Fryer at 375°F.
2. Take a baking dish small enough to fit inside the fryer and spritz it with cooking spray.
3. Combine all the ingredients to coat the tofu completely and allow the marinade to absorb for half an hour.
4. Transfer the tofu to the baking dish, then cook for 15 minutes. Flip the tofu over and cook for another 15 minute on the other side.

55. Parmesan Beef Mix

Servings: 4
Cooking Time: 20 Minutes
Ingredients:
- 14 ounces beef, cubed
- 7 ounces keto tomato sauce
- 1 tablespoon chives, chopped
- 2 tablespoons parmesan cheese, grated
- 1 tablespoon oregano, chopped
- 1 tablespoon olive oil
- Salt and black pepper to the taste

Directions:
1. Grease a pan that fits the air fryer with the oil and mix all the ingredients except the parmesan. Sprinkle the parmesan on top, put the pan in the machine and cook at 380

degrees F for 20 minutes. Divide between plates and serve for lunch.

56. Christmas Brussels Sprouts

Servings: 2
Cooking Time: 20 Minutes
Ingredients:
- 2 cups Brussels sprouts, halved
- 1 tbsp. olive oil
- 1 tbsp. balsamic vinegar
- 1 tbsp. maple syrup
- ¼ tsp. sea salt

Directions:
1. Pre-heat the Air Fryer at 375°F.
2. Evenly coat the Brussels sprouts with the olive oil, balsamic vinegar, maple syrup, and salt.
3. Transfer to the basket of your fryer and cook for 5 minutes. Give the basket a good shake, turn the heat up to 400°F and continue to cook for another 8 minutes.

57. Grilled Ham & Cheese

Servings: 2
Cooking Time: 30 Minutes
Ingredients:
- 3 low-carb buns
- 4 slices medium-cut deli ham
- 1 tbsp salted butter
- 1 oz. flour
- 3 slices cheddar cheese
- 3 slices muenster cheese

Directions:
1. Bread:
2. Preheat your fryer to 350°F/175°C.
3. Mix the flour, salt and baking powder in a bowl. Put to the side.
4. Add in the butter and coconut oil to a skillet.
5. Melt for 20 seconds and pour into another bowl.

6. In this bowl, mix in the dough.
7. Scramble two eggs. Add to the dough.
8. Add ½ tablespoon of coconut flour to thicken, and place evenly into a cupcake tray. Fill about ¾ inch.
9. Bake for 20 minutes until browned.
10. Allow to cool for 15 minutes and cut each in half for the buns.
11. Sandwich:
12. Fry the deli meat in a skillet on a high heat.
13. Put the ham and cheese between the buns.
14. Heat the butter on medium high.
15. When brown, turn to low and add the dough to pan.
16. Press down with a weight until you smell burning, then flip to crisp both sides.
17. Enjoy!

58. Cheddar Beef Chili

Servings: 2
Cooking Time: 20 Minutes
Ingredients:
- 1 cup ground beef
- ¼ cup Cheddar cheese, shredded
- ¼ cup green beans, trimmed and halved
- ¼ cup spring onion, diced
- 1 teaspoon fresh cilantro, chopped
- 2 chili pepper, chopped
- 1 teaspoon ghee
- 1 tablespoon keto tomato sauce
- ½ cup chicken broth
- ½ teaspoon salt
- ¼ teaspoon garlic powder

Directions:
1. Put ghee in the skillet and melt it. Put the ground beef in the skillet. Add spring onion, garlic powder, and salt. Stir the ground beef mixture and cook

it over the medium heat for 5 minutes. Then transfer the mixture in the air fryer pan. Add tomato sauce and stir until homogenous. Add chicken broth, chili peppers, and cilantro. Then add green beans and cilantro. Mix up the chili gently and top with Cheddar cheese. Preheat the air fryer to 390F. Put the pan with chili con carne in the air fryer and cook it for 10 minutes.

59. Pepperoni Pizza

Servings: 3
Cooking Time: 15 Minutes
Ingredients:
- 3 portobello mushroom caps, cleaned and scooped
- 3 tbsp. olive oil
- 3 tbsp. tomato sauce
- 3 tbsp. mozzarella, shredded
- 12 slices pepperoni
- 1 pinch salt
- 1 pinch dried Italian seasonings

Directions:
1. Pre-heat the Air Fryer to 330°F.
2. Season both sides of the portobello mushrooms with a drizzle of olive oil, then sprinkle salt and the Italian seasonings on the insides.
3. With a knife, spread the tomato sauce evenly over the mushroom, before adding the mozzarella on top.
4. Put the portobello in the cooking basket and place in the Air Fryer.
5. Cook for 1 minute, before taking the cooking basket out of the fryer and putting the pepperoni slices on top.
6. Cook for another 3 to 5 minutes. Garnish with freshly grated parmesan cheese and crushed red pepper flakes and serve.

60. Leeks Stew

Servings: 4
Cooking Time: 20 Minutes
Ingredients:
- 2 big eggplants, roughly cubed
- 1 cup veggie stock
- 3 leeks, sliced
- 2 tablespoons olive oil
- 1 tablespoon hot sauce
- 1 tablespoon sweet paprika
- 1 tablespoon keto tomato sauce
- Salt and black pepper to the taste
- ½ bunch cilantro, chopped
- 2 garlic cloves, minced

Directions:
1. In a pan that fits the air fryer, mix all the ingredients, toss, introduce in the fryer and cook at 380 degrees F for 20 minutes. Divide the stew into bowls and serve for lunch.

61. Beef And Sauce

Servings: 4
Cooking Time: 20 Minutes
Ingredients:
- 1 pound lean beef meat, cubed and browned
- 2 garlic cloves, minced
- Salt and black pepper to the taste
- Cooking spray
- 16 ounces keto tomato sauce

Directions:
1. Preheat the Air Fryer at 400 degrees F, add the pan inside, grease it with cooking spray, add the meat and all the other ingredients, toss and cook for 20 minutes. Divide into bowls and serve for lunch.

62. Veggie Pizza

Servings: 4
Cooking Time: 15 Minutes
Ingredients:
- 8 bacon slices
- ¼ cup black olives, sliced
- ¼ cup scallions, sliced
- 1 green bell pepper, sliced
- 1 cup Mozzarella, shredded
- 1 tablespoon keto tomato sauce
- ½ teaspoon dried basil
- ½ teaspoon sesame oil

Directions:
1. Line the air fryer pan with baking paper. Then make the layer of the sliced bacon in the pan and sprinkle gently with sesame oil. Preheat the air fryer to 400F. Place the pan with the bacon in the air fryer basket and cook it for 9 minutes at 400F. After this, sprinkle the bacon with keto tomato sauce and top with Mozzarella. Then add bell pepper, spring onions, and black olives. Sprinkle the pizza with dried basil and cook for 6 minutes at 400F.

VEGETABLE & SIDE DISHES

63. Sweet Mixed Nuts

Servings:5
Cooking Time: 25 Minutes
Ingredients:

- ½ cup walnuts
- ½ cup almonds
- A pinch cayenne pepper
- 2 tbsp sugar
- 2 tbsp egg whites
- 2 tsp cinnamon
- Cooking spray

Directions:

1. Add pepper, sugar, and cinnamon to a bowl and mix well; set aside. In another bowl, mix pecans, walnuts, almonds, and egg whites. Add the spice mixture to the nuts and mix. Grease the fryer basket with cooking spray. Pour in the nuts, and cook for 10 minutes. Stir the nuts using a wooden vessel, and cook for further for 10 minutes. Pour the nuts in the bowl. Let cool before serving.

64. Roasted Beet Salad

Servings: 2
Cooking Time: 20 Minutes + Chilling Time
Ingredients:

- 2 medium-sized beets, peeled and cut into wedges
- 2 tablespoons extra virgin olive oil
- 1 tablespoon balsamic vinegar
- 1 teaspoon yellow mustard
- 1 garlic clove, minced
- 1/4 teaspoon cumin powder
- Coarse sea salt and ground black pepper, to taste
- 1 tablespoon fresh parsley leaves, roughly chopped

Directions:

1. Place the beets in a single layer in the lightly greased cooking basket.
2. Cook at 370 degrees F for 13 minutes, shaking the basket halfway through the cooking time.
3. Let it cool to room temperature; toss the beets with the remaining ingredients. Serve well chilled. Enjoy!

65. Endives And Rice Mix

Servings: 4
Cooking Time: 20 Minutes
Ingredients:

- 2 scallions, chopped
- 3 garlic cloves, minced
- 1 tablespoon olive oil
- Salt and black pepper to taste
- ½ cup white rice
- 1 cup veggie stock
- 1 teaspoon chili sauce
- 4 endives, trimmed and shredded

Directions:

1. Take the oil and grease a pan that fits your air fryer.
2. Add all other ingredients and toss.
3. Place the pan in the air fryer and cook at 365 degrees F for 20 minutes.
4. Divide everything between plates and serve as a side dish.

66. Japanese Tempura Bowl

Servings: 3
Cooking Time: 20 Minutes
Ingredients:

- 1 cup all-purpose flour
- Kosher salt and ground black pepper, to taste
- 1/2 teaspoon paprika
- 2 eggs
- 3 tablespoons soda water
- 1 cup panko crumbs

- 2 tablespoons olive oil
- 1 cup green beans
- 1 onion, cut into rings
- 1 zucchini, cut into slices
- 2 tablespoons soy sauce
- 1 tablespoon mirin
- 1 teaspoon dashi granules

Directions:

1. In a shallow bowl, mix the flour, salt, black pepper, and paprika. In a separate bowl, whisk the eggs and soda water. In a third shallow bowl, combine the panko crumbs with olive oil.
2. Dip the vegetables in flour mixture, then in the egg mixture; lastly, roll over the panko mixture to coat evenly.
3. Cook in the preheated Air Fryer at 400 degrees F for 10 minutes, shaking the basket halfway through the cooking time. Work in batches until the vegetables are crispy and golden brown.
4. Then, make the sauce by whisking the soy sauce, mirin, and dashi granules. Bon appétit!

67. Creamy Spinach

Servings: 6
Cooking Time: 16 Minutes
Ingredients:

- 1 lb fresh spinach
- 6 oz gouda cheese, shredded
- 8 oz cream cheese
- 1 tsp garlic powder
- 1 tbsp onion, minced
- Pepper
- Salt

Directions:

1. Preheat the air fryer to 370 F.
2. Spray air fryer baking dish with cooking spray and set aside.

3. Spray a large pan with cooking spray and heat over medium heat.
4. Add spinach to the pan and cook until wilted.
5. Add cream cheese, garlic powder, and onion and stir until cheese is melted.
6. Remove pan from heat and add Gouda cheese and season with pepper and salt.
7. Transfer spinach mixture to the prepared baking dish and place into the air fryer.
8. Cook for 16 minutes.
9. Serve and enjoy.

68. Easy Sweet Potato Hash Browns

Servings: 2
Cooking Time: 50 Minutes
Ingredients:

- 1 pound sweet potatoes, peeled and grated
- 2 eggs, whisked
- 1/4 cup scallions, chopped
- 1 teaspoon fresh garlic, minced
- Sea salt and ground black pepper, to taste
- 1/4 teaspoon ground allspice
- 1/2 teaspoon cinnamon
- 1 tablespoon peanut oil

Directions:

1. Allow the sweet potatoes to soak for 25 minutes in cold water. Drain the water; dry the sweet potatoes with a kitchen towel.
2. Add the remaining ingredients and stir to combine well.
3. Cook in the preheated Air Fryer at 395 degrees F for 20 minutes. Shake the basket once or twice. Serve with ketchup.

69. Turkey Garlic Potatoes

Servings: 2

Cooking Time: 45 Minutes

Ingredients:

- 3 unsmoked turkey strips
- 6 small potatoes
- 1 tsp. garlic, minced
- 2 tsp. olive oil
- Salt to taste
- Pepper to taste

Directions:

1. Peel the potatoes and cube them finely.
2. Coat in 1 teaspoon of oil and cook in the Air Fryer for 10 minutes at 350°F.
3. In a separate bowl, slice the turkey finely and combine with the garlic, oil, salt and pepper. Pour the potatoes into the bowl and mix well.
4. Lay the mixture on some silver aluminum foil, transfer to the fryer and cook for about 10 minutes.
5. Serve with raita.

70. Pumpkin Wedges

Servings:3
Cooking Time: 30 Minutes

Ingredients:

- 1 tbsp paprika
- 1 whole lime, squeezed
- 1 cup paleo dressing
- 1 tbsp balsamic vinegar
- Salt and pepper to taste
- 1 tsp turmeric

Directions:

1. Preheat your air fryer to 360 F. Add the pumpkin wedges in your air fryer's cooking basket, and cook for 20 minutes. In a mixing bowl, mix lime juice, vinegar, turmeric, salt, pepper and paprika to form a marinade. Pour the marinade over pumpkin, and cook for 5 more minutes.

71. Italian-style Eggplant With Mozzarella Cheese

Servings: 4
Cooking Time: 45 Minutes

Ingredients:

- 1 pound eggplant, sliced
- 1 tablespoon sea salt
- 1/2 cup Romano cheese, preferably freshly grated
- Sea salt and cracked black pepper, to taste
- 1 egg, whisked
- 4 ounces pork rinds
- 1/2 cup mozzarella cheese, grated
- 2 tablespoons fresh Italian parsley, roughly chopped

Directions:

1. Toss the eggplant with 1 tablespoon of salt and let it stand for 30 minutes. Drain and rinse.
2. Mix the cheese, salt, and black pepper in a bowl. Then, add the whisked egg.
3. Dip the eggplant slices in the batter and press to coat on all sides. Roll them over pork rinds. Transfer to the lightly greased Air Fryer basket.
4. Cook at 370 degrees F for 7 to 9 minutes. Turn each slice over and top with the mozzarella. Cook an additional 2 minutes or until the cheese melts.
5. Serve garnished with fresh Italian parsley. Bon appétit!

72. Balsamic Garlic Kale

Servings: 6
Cooking Time: 12 Minutes

Ingredients:

- 2 tablespoons olive oil
- 3 garlic cloves, minced
- 2 and ½ pounds kale leaves
- Salt and black pepper to the taste

- 2 tablespoons balsamic vinegar

Directions:

1. In a pan that fits the air fryer, combine all the ingredients and toss. Put the pan in your air fryer and cook at 300 degrees F for 12 minutes. Divide between plates and serve.

73. Spicy Kale

Servings: 4

Cooking Time: 10 Minutes

Ingredients:

- 1 pound kale, torn
- 1 tablespoon olive oil
- 1 teaspoon hot paprika
- A pinch of salt and black pepper
- 2 tablespoons oregano, chopped

Directions:

1. In a pan that fits the air fryer, combine all the ingredients and toss. Put the pan in the air fryer and cook at 380 degrees F for 10 minutes. Divide between plates and serve.

74. Sweet Corn Fritters

Servings: 4

Cooking Time: 20 Minutes

Ingredients:

- 1 medium-sized carrot, grated
- 1 yellow onion, finely chopped
- 4 oz. canned sweet corn kernels, drained
- 1 tsp. sea salt flakes
- 1 heaping tbsp. fresh cilantro, chopped
- 1 medium-sized egg, whisked
- 2 tbsp. plain milk
- 1 cup of Parmesan cheese, grated
- ¼ cup flour
- ⅓ tsp. baking powder
- ⅓ tsp. sugar

Directions:

1. Place the grated carrot in a colander and press down to squeeze out any excess moisture. Dry it with a paper towel.
2. Combine the carrots with the remaining ingredients.
3. Mold 1 tablespoon of the mixture into a ball and press it down with your hand or a spoon to flatten it. Repeat until the rest of the mixture is used up.
4. Spritz the balls with cooking spray.
5. Arrange in the basket of your Air Fryer, taking care not to overlap any balls. Cook at 350°F for 8 to 11 minutes or until they're firm.
6. Serve warm.

75. Air-fried Cheesy Broccoli With Garlic

Servings:2

Cooking Time: 25 Minutes

Ingredients:

- 1 egg white
- 1 garlic clove, grated
- Salt and black pepper to taste
- ½ lb broccoli florets
- ⅓ cup grated Parmesan cheese

Directions:

1. In a bowl, whisk together the butter, egg, garlic, salt, and black pepper. Toss in broccoli to coat well. Top with Parmesan cheese and; toss to coat. Arrange broccoli in a single layer in the air fryer, without overcrowding. Cook for 10 minutes at 360 F. Remove to a plate and sprinkle with Parmesan cheese.

76. Green Beans And Tomatoes Recipe

Servings: 4

Cooking Time:25 Minutes

Ingredients:

- 1-pint cherry tomatoes

- 2 tbsp. olive oil
- 1 lb. green beans
- Salt and black pepper to the taste

Directions:

1. In a bowl; mix cherry tomatoes with green beans, olive oil, salt and pepper, toss, transfer to your air fryer and cook at 400 °F, for 15 minutes. Divide among plates and serve right away

77. Cauliflower Patties

Servings: 2
Cooking Time: 10 Minutes
Ingredients:

- ¼ cup cauliflower, shredded
- 1 egg yolk
- ½ teaspoon ground turmeric
- ¼ teaspoon onion powder
- ¼ teaspoon salt
- 2 oz Cheddar cheese, shredded
- ¼ teaspoon baking powder
- 1 teaspoon heavy cream
- 1 tablespoon coconut flakes
- Cooking spray

Directions:

1. Squeeze the shredded cauliflower and put it in the bowl. Add egg yolk, ground turmeric, onion powder, baking powder, salt, heavy cream, and coconut flakes. Then melt Cheddar cheese and add it in the cauliflower mixture. Stir the ingredients until you get the smooth mass. After this, make the medium size cauliflower patties. Preheat the air fryer to 365F. Spray the air fryer basket with cooking spray and put the patties inside. Cook them for 5 minutes from each side.

78. Broccoli Puree

Servings: 4

Cooking Time: 20 Minutes
Ingredients:

- 20 ounces broccoli florets
- A drizzle of olive oil
- 4 tablespoons basil, chopped
- 3 ounces butter, melted
- 1 garlic clove, minced
- A pinch of salt and black pepper

Directions:

1. In a bowl, mix the broccoli with the oil, salt and pepper, toss and transfer to your air fryer's basket. Cook at 380 degrees F for 20 minutes, cool the broccoli down and put it in a blender. Add the rest of the ingredients, pulse, divide the mash between plates and serve as a side dish.

79. Crispy Bacon With Butterbean Dip

Servings:2
Cooking Time: 10 Minutes
Ingredients:

- 1 tbsp chives
- 3 ½ oz feta
- Pepper to taste
- 1 tsp olive oil
- 3 ½ oz bacon, sliced

Directions:

1. Preheat your air fryer to 340 F. Blend beans, oil and pepper using a blender. Arrange bacon slices on your air fryer's cooking basket. Sprinkle chives on top and cook for 10 minutes. Add feta cheese to the butter bean blend and stir. Serve bacon with the dip.

80. Crispy Parmesan Asparagus

Servings: 4
Cooking Time: 20 Minutes
Ingredients:

- 2 eggs

- 1 teaspoon Dijon mustard
- 1 cup Parmesan cheese, grated
- 1 cup bread crumbs
- Sea salt and ground black pepper, to taste
- 18 asparagus spears, trimmed
- 1/2 cup sour cream

Directions:
1. Start by preheating your Air Fryer to 400 degrees F.
2. In a shallow bowl, whisk the eggs and mustard. In another shallow bowl, combine the Parmesan cheese, breadcrumbs, salt, and black pepper.
3. Dip the asparagus spears in the egg mixture, then in the parmesan mixture; press to adhere.
4. Cook for 5 minutes; work in three batches. Serve with sour cream on the side. Enjoy!

81. Ghee Savoy Cabbage

Servings: 4
Cooking Time: 15 Minutes
Ingredients:
- 1 Savoy cabbage head, shredded
- Salt and black pepper to the taste
- 1 and ½ tablespoons ghee, melted
- ¼ cup coconut cream
- 1 tablespoon dill, chopped

Directions:
1. In a pan that fits the air fryer, combine all the ingredients except the coconut cream, toss, put the pan in the air fryer and cook at 390 degrees F for 10 minutes. Add the cream, toss, cook for 5 minutes more, divide between plates and serve.

82. Kabocha Fries

Servings: 2
Cooking Time: 11 Minutes

Ingredients:
- 6 oz Kabocha squash, peeled
- ½ teaspoon olive oil
- ½ teaspoon salt

Directions:
1. Cut the Kabocha squash into the shape of the French fries and sprinkle with olive oil. Preheat the air fryer to 390F. Put the Kabocha squash fries in the air fryer basket and cook them for 5 minutes. Then shake them well and cook for 6 minutes more. Sprinkle the cooked Kabocha fries with salt and mix up well.

83. Spinach Mash

Servings: 4
Cooking Time: 13 Minutes
Ingredients:
- 3 cups spinach, chopped
- ½ cup Mozzarella, shredded
- 4 bacon slices, chopped
- 1 teaspoon butter
- 1 cup heavy cream
- ½ teaspoon salt
- ½ jalapeno pepper, chopped

Directions:
1. Place the bacon in the air fryer and cook it for 8 minutes at 400F. Stir it from time to time with the help of the spatula. After this, put the cooked bacon in the air fryer casserole mold. Add heavy cream spinach, jalapeno pepper, salt, butter, and Mozzarella. Stir it gently. Cook the mash for 5 minutes at 400F. Then stir the spinach mash carefully with the help of the spoon.

84. Quick Rutabaga Chips

Servings:1
Cooking Time: 20 Minutes

Ingredients:
- 1 tsp olive oil
- 1 tsp soy sauce
- Salt to taste

Directions:
1. Preheat air fryer to 400 F. In a bowl, mix oil, soy sauce, and salt. Add rutabaga pieces and allow to stand for 5 minutes. Cook in your air fryer for 5 minutes, tossing once halfway through cooking.

85. Garlic Stuffed Mushrooms

Servings: 4
Cooking Time: 25 Minutes
Ingredients:
- 6 small mushrooms
- 1 oz. onion, peeled and diced
- 1 tbsp. friendly bread crumbs
- 1 tbsp. olive oil
- 1 tsp. garlic, pureed
- 1 tsp. parsley
- Salt and pepper to taste

Directions:
1. Combine the bread crumbs, oil, onion, parsley, salt, pepper and garlic in a bowl. Cut out the mushrooms' stalks and stuff each cap with the crumb mixture.
2. Cook in the Air Fryer for 10 minutes at 350°F.
3. Serve with a side of mayo dip.

86. Easy Sweet Potato Bake

Servings: 3
Cooking Time: 35 Minutes
Ingredients:
- 1 stick butter, melted
- 1 pound sweet potatoes, mashed
- 2 tablespoons honey
- 2 eggs, beaten
- 1/3 cup coconut milk
- 1/4 cup flour
- 1/2 cup fresh breadcrumbs

Directions:
1. Start by preheating your Air Fryer to 325 degrees F.
2. Spritz a casserole dish with cooking oil.
3. In a mixing bowl, combine all ingredients, except for the breadcrumbs and 1 tablespoon of butter. Spoon the mixture into the prepared casserole dish.
4. Top with the breadcrumbs and brush the top with the remaining 1 tablespoon of butter. Bake in the preheated Air Fryer for 30 minutes. Bon appétit!

87. Butter Cabbage

Servings: 4
Cooking Time: 20 Minutes
Ingredients:
- 2 ounces butter, melted
- 1 green cabbage head, shredded
- 1 and ½ cups heavy cream
- ¼ cup parsley, chopped
- 1 tablespoon sweet paprika
- 1 teaspoon lemon zest, grated

Directions:
1. Heat up a pan that fits the air fryer with the butter, add the cabbage and sauté for 5 minutes. Add the remaining ingredients, toss, put the pan in the air fryer and cook at 380 degrees F for 15 minutes. Divide between plates and serve as a side dish.

88. Rustic Roasted Green Beans

Servings: 4
Cooking Time: 10 Minutes + Chilling Time
Ingredients:

- 3/4 pound trimmed green beans, cut into bite-sized pieces
- Salt and freshly cracked mixed pepper, to taste
- 1 shallot, thinly sliced
- 1 tablespoon lime juice
- 1 tablespoon champagne vinegar
- 1/4 cup extra-virgin olive oil
- 1/2 teaspoon mustard seeds
- 1/2 teaspoon celery seeds
- 1 tablespoon fresh basil leaves, chopped
- 1 tablespoon fresh parsley leaves
- 1 cup goat cheese, crumbled

Directions:
1. Toss the green beans with salt and pepper in a lightly greased Air Fryer basket.
2. Cook in the preheated Air Fryer at 400 degrees F for 5 minutes or until tender.
3. Add the shallots and gently stir to combine.
4. In a mixing bowl, whisk the lime juice, vinegar, olive oil, and spices. Dress the salad and top with the goat cheese. Serve at room temperature or chilled. Enjoy!

89. Lime Green Beans And Sauce

Servings: 4
Cooking Time: 8 Minutes
Ingredients:
- 1 pound green beans, trimmed
- 1 tablespoon lime juice
- A pinch of salt and black pepper
- 2 tablespoons ghee, melted
- 1 teaspoon chili powder

Directions:
1. In a bowl, mix the ghee with the rest of the ingredients except the green beans and whisk really well. Mix the

green beans with the lime sauce, toss, put them in your air fryer's basket and cook at 400 degrees F for 8 minutes. Serve right away.

90. Asian Cauliflower Rice With Eggs

Servings: 4
Cooking Time: 20 Minutes
Ingredients:
- 2 cups cauliflower, food-processed into rice-like particles
- 2 tablespoons peanut oil
- 1/2 cup scallions, chopped
- 2 bell pepper, chopped
- 4 eggs, beaten
- Sea salt and ground black pepper, to taste
- 1/2 teaspoon granulated garlic

Directions:
1. Grease a baking pan with nonstick cooking spray.
2. Add the cauliflower rice and the other ingredients to the baking pan.
3. Cook at 400 degrees F for 12 minutes, checking occasionally to ensure even cooking. Enjoy!

91. Spinach Salad

Servings: 4
Cooking Time: 10 Minutes
Ingredients:
- 1 pound baby spinach
- Salt and black pepper to the taste
- 1 tablespoon mustard
- Cooking spray
- ¼ cup apple cider vinegar
- 1 tablespoon chives, chopped

Directions:
1. Grease a pan that fits your air fryer with cooking spray, combine all the ingredients, introduce the pan in the fryer and cook at 350 degrees F for

10 minutes. Divide between plates and serve as a side dish.

92. Simple Cauliflower Bars

Servings: 12
Cooking Time:35 Minutes
Ingredients:
- 1 big cauliflower head; florets separated
- 1 tsp. Italian seasoning
- 1/2 cup mozzarella; shredded
- 1/4 cup egg whites
- Salt and black pepper to the taste

Directions:
1. Put cauliflower florets in your food processor; pulse well, spread on a lined baking sheet that fits your air fryer, introduce in the fryer and cook at 360 °F, for 10 minutes.
2. Transfer cauliflower to a bowl; add salt, pepper, cheese, egg whites and Italian seasoning; stir really well, spread this into a rectangle pan that fits your air fryer; press well, introduce in the fryer and cook at 360 °F, for 15 minutes more. Cut into

12 bars, arrange them on a platter and serve as a snack

93. Potatoes And Special Tomato Sauce Recipe

Servings: 4
Cooking Time:26 Minutes
Ingredients:
- 2 lbs. potatoes; cubed
- 4 garlic cloves; minced
- 1 yellow onion; chopped.
- 1 cup tomato sauce
- 1/2 tsp. oregano; dried
- 1/2 tsp. parsley; dried
- 2 tbsp. basil; chopped
- 2 tbsp. olive oil

Directions:
1. Heat up a pan that fits your air fryer with the oil over medium heat, add onion; stir and cook for 1-2 minutes.
2. Add garlic, potatoes, parsley, tomato sauce and oregano; stir, introduce in your air fryer and cook at 370 °F and cook for 16 minutes. Add basil, toss everything, divide among plates and serve

VEGAN & VEGETARIAN RECIPES

94. Paprika Vegetable Kabobs

Servings: 4
Cooking Time: 20 Minutes
Ingredients:
- 1 celery, cut into thick slices
- 1 parsnip, cut into thick slices
- 1 fennel bulb, diced
- 1 teaspoon whole grain mustard
- 2 cloves garlic, pressed
- 1 red onion, cut into wedges
- 2 tablespoons dry white wine
- 1/4 cup sesame oil
- 1 teaspoon sea salt flakes
- 1/2 teaspoon ground black pepper
- 1 teaspoon smoked paprika

Directions:
1. Place all of the above ingredients in a mixing dish; toss to coat well. Alternately thread vegetables onto the bamboo skewers.
2. Cook on the Air Fryer grill pan for 15 minutes at 380 degrees F. Flip them over halfway through the cooking time.
3. Taste, adjust the seasonings and serve warm.

95. Refreshingly Zesty Broccoli

Servings:4
Cooking Time:15 Minutes
Ingredients:
- 1 tablespoon butter
- 1 large head broccoli, cut into bite-sized pieces
- 1 tablespoon white sesame seeds
- 2 tablespoons vegetable stock
- 1 tablespoon fresh lemon juice
- 3 garlic cloves, chopped
- ½ teaspoon fresh lemon zest, grated finely

- ½ teaspoon red pepper flakes, crushed

Directions:
1. Preheat the Air fryer to 355 °F and grease an Air fryer pan.
2. Mix butter, vegetable stock and lemon juice in the Air fryer pan.
3. Transfer into the Air fryer and cook for about 2 minutes.
4. Stir in garlic and broccoli and cook for about 14 minutes.
5. Add sesame seeds, lemon zest and red pepper flakes and cook for 5 minutes.
6. Dish out and serve warm.

96. Cauliflower Salad

Servings:4
Cooking Time:10 Minutes
Ingredients:
- ¼ cup golden raisins
- 1 cup boiling water
- 1 head cauliflower, cut into small florets
- ¼ cup pecans, toasted and chopped
- 2 tablespoons fresh mint leaves, chopped
- ¼ cup olive oil
- 1 tablespoon curry powder
- Salt, to taste
- For Dressing
- 1 cup mayonnaise
- 2 tablespoons sugar
- 1 tablespoon fresh lemon juice

Directions:
1. Preheat the Air fryer to 390 °F and grease an Air fryer basket.
2. Mix the cauliflower, curry powder, salt, and olive oil in a bowl and toss to coat well.

3. Arrange the cauliflower florets in the Air fryer basket and cook for about 10 minutes.
4. Dish out the cauliflower florets in a serving bowl and keep aside to cool.
5. Meanwhile, add the raisins in boiling water in a bowl for about 20 minutes.
6. Drain the raisins well and mix with the cauliflower florets.
7. Mix all the ingredients for dressing in a bowl and pour over the salad.
8. Toss to coat well and serve immediately.

97. Italian-style Risi E Bisi

Servings: 4
Cooking Time: 20 Minutes
Ingredients:
- 2 cups brown rice
- 4 cups water
- 1/2 cup frozen green peas
- 3 tablespoons soy sauce
- 1 tablespoon olive oil
- 1 cup brown mushrooms, sliced
- 2 garlic cloves, minced
- 1 small-sized onion, chopped
- 1 tablespoon fresh parsley, chopped

Directions:
1. Heat the brown rice and water in a pot over high heat. Bring it to a boil; turn the stove down to simmer and cook for 35 minutes. Allow your rice to cool completely.
2. Transfer the cold cooked rice to the lightly greased Air Fryer pan. Add the remaining ingredients and stir to combine.
3. Cook in the preheated Air Fryer at 360 degrees F for 18 to 22 minutes. Serve warm.

98. Minty Green Beans With Shallots

Servings:6
Cooking Time: 25 Minutes
Ingredients:
- 1 tablespoon fresh mint, chopped
- 1 tablespoon sesame seeds, toasted
- 1 tablespoon vegetable oil
- 1 teaspoon soy sauce
- 1-pound fresh green beans, trimmed
- 2 large shallots, sliced
- 2 tablespoons fresh basil, chopped
- 2 tablespoons pine nuts

Directions:
1. Preheat the air fryer to 330 °F.
2. Place the grill pan accessory in the air fryer.
3. In a mixing bowl, combine the green beans, shallots, vegetable oil, and soy sauce.
4. Dump in the air fryer and cook for 25 minutes.
5. Once cooked, garnish with basil, mints, sesame seeds, and pine nuts.

99. Mediterranean Falafel With Tzatziki

Servings: 4
Cooking Time: 30 Minutes
Ingredients:
- For the Falafel:
- 2 cups cauliflower, grated
- 1/4 teaspoon baking powder
- 1/3 cup warm water
- 1/2 teaspoon salt
- 1 tablespoon coriander leaves, finely chopped
- 2 tablespoons fresh lemon juice
- Vegan Tzatziki:
- 1 cup plain Greek yogurt
- 2 tablespoons lime juice, freshly squeezed
- 1/4 teaspoon ground black pepper, or more to taste

- 1/3 teaspoon sea salt flakes
- 2 tablespoons extra-virgin olive oil
- 2 tablespoons chopped fresh dill
- 1 clove garlic, pressed
- 1/2 fresh cucumber, grated

Directions:

1. In a bowl, thoroughly combine all the ingredients for the falafel. Allow the mixture to stay for approximately 10 minutes.
2. Now, air-fry at 390 degrees F for 15 minutes; make sure to flip them over halfway through the cooking time.
3. To make Greek tzatziki, blend all ingredients in your food processor.
4. Serve warm falafel with chilled tzatziki. Enjoy!

100. Winter Squash And Tomato Bake

Servings: 4
Cooking Time: 30 Minutes
Ingredients:

- Cashew Cream:
- 1/2 cup sunflower seeds, soaked overnight, rinsed and drained
- 1/4 cup lime juice
- Sea salt, to taste
- 2 teaspoons nutritional yeast
- 1 tablespoon tahini
- 1/2 cup water
- Squash:
- 1 pound winter squash, peeled and sliced
- 2 tablespoons olive oil
- Sea salt and ground black pepper, to taste
- Sauce:
- 2 tablespoons olive oil
- 2 ripe tomatoes, crushed
- 6 ounces spinach, torn into small pieces
- 2 garlic cloves, minced

- 1 cup vegetable broth
- 1/2 teaspoon dried rosemary
- 1/2 teaspoon dried basil

Directions:

1. Mix the ingredients for the cashew cream in your food processor until creamy and uniform. Reserve.
2. Place the squash slices in the lightly greased casserole dish. Add the olive oil, salt, and black pepper.
3. Mix all the ingredients for the sauce. Pour the sauce over the vegetables. Bake in the preheated Air Fryer at 390 degrees F for 15 minutes.
4. Top with the cashew cream and bake an additional 5 minutes or until everything is thoroughly heated.
5. Transfer to a wire rack to cool slightly before sling and serving.

101. Rich And Easy Vegetable Croquettes

Servings: 4
Cooking Time: 15 Minutes
Ingredients:

- 1/2 pound broccoli florets
- 1 tablespoon ground flaxseeds
- 1 yellow onion, finely chopped
- 1 bell pepper, seeded and chopped
- 2 garlic cloves, pressed
- 1 teaspoon turmeric powder
- 1/2 teaspoon ground cumin
- 1/2 cup almond flour
- 1/2 cup parmesan cheese
- 2 eggs, whisked
- Salt and ground black pepper, to taste
- 2 tablespoons olive oil

Directions:

1. Blanch the broccoli in salted boiling water until al dente, about 3 to 4 minutes. Drain well and transfer to a mixing bowl; mash the broccoli

florets with the remaining ingredients.

2. Form the mixture into patties and place them in the lightly greased Air Fryer basket.
3. Cook at 400 degrees F for 6 minutes, turning them over halfway through the cooking time; work in batches.
4. Serve warm with mayonnaise. Enjoy!

102.Veggie Fingers With Monterey Jack Cheese

Servings: 4
Cooking Time: 20 Minutes
Ingredients:
- 10 ounces cauliflower
- 1/4 cup almond flour
- 1 ½ teaspoons soy sauce
- Salt and freshly ground black pepper, to taste
- 1 teaspoon cayenne pepper
- 1 cup parmesan cheese, grated
- 3/4 teaspoon dried dill weed
- 1 tablespoon olive oil

Directions:
1. Firstly, pulse the cauliflower in your food processor; transfer them to a bowl and add 1/4 cup almond flour, soy sauce, salt, black pepper, and cayenne pepper.
2. Roll the mixture into veggie fingers shape. In another bowl, place grated parmesan cheese and dried dill.
3. Now, coat the veggie fingers with the parmesan mixture, covering completely. Drizzle veggie fingers with olive oil.
4. Air-fry for 15 minutes at 350 degrees F; turn them over once or twice during the cooking time. Eat with your favorite sauce. Enjoy!

103.Vegetable Croquettes

Servings:3
Cooking Time: 30 Minutes
Ingredients:
- 2 cups water
- 1 ¼ cups milk
- Salt to taste
- 2 tsp + 3 tsp butter
- 2 tsp olive oil
- 2 red peppers, chopped
- ½ cup baby spinach, chopped
- 3 mushrooms, chopped
- 1/6 broccoli florets, chopped
- 1/6 cup sliced green onion
- ½ red onion, chopped
- 2 cloves garlic, minced
- 1 medium carrot, grated
- ⅓ cup flour
- 2 tbsp cornstarch
- 1 ½ cups breadcrumbs
- Cooking spray

Directions:
1. Place the potatoes in a pot, add the water, and bring it to boil over medium heat on a stovetop. Boil until tender and mashable. Drain the potatoes through a sieve and place them in a bowl.
2. Add the 2 teaspoons of butter, 1 cup of milk, and salt. Use a potato masher to mash well; set aside.
3. Place a skillet over medium heat and melt the remaining butter. Add onion, garlic, red peppers, broccoli, and mushrooms; stir-fry for 2 minutes. Add green onion and spinach, and cook until the spinach wilts.
4. Season with salt and stir. Turn the heat off and pour the veggie mixture into the potato mash. Use the potato masher to mash the veggies into the

potatoes; allow cooling. Using your hands, form oblong balls of the mixture and place them on a baking sheet in a single layer. Refrigerate for 30 minutes.

5. In 3 separate bowls, add breadcrumbs in one, flour in another, and cornstarch, remaining milk and salt in a third bowl. Mix cornstarch, salt and 1 tbsp of water. Remove the patties from the fridge.

6. Preheat the fryer to 390 F. Dredge each veggie mold in flour, then in the cornstarch mixture, and then in the breadcrumbs. Place the patties in batches in a single layer in the basket without overlapping. Spray with olive oil and cook for 2 minutes. Flip, spray them with cooking spray and cook for more 3 minutes. Remove to a wire rack and serve with tomato sauce.

104.Cauliflower, Broccoli And Chickpea Salad

Servings: 4
Cooking Time: 20 Minutes + Chilling Time
Ingredients:
- 1/2 pound cauliflower florets
- 1/2 pound broccoli florets
- Sea salt, to taste
- 1/2 teaspoon red pepper flakes
- 2 tablespoons soy sauce
- 2 tablespoons cider vinegar
- 1 teaspoon Dijon mustard
- 2 tablespoons extra-virgin olive oil
- 1 cup canned or cooked chickpeas, drained
- 1 avocado, pitted, peeled and sliced
- 1 small sized onion, peeled and sliced
- 1 garlic clove, minced
- 2 cups arugula

- 2 tablespoons sesame seeds, lightly toasted

Directions:
1. Start by preheating your Air Fryer to 400 degrees F.
2. Brush the cauliflower and broccoli florets with cooking spray.
3. Cook for 12 minutes, shaking the cooking basket halfway through the cooking time. Season with salt and red pepper.
4. In a mixing dish, whisk the soy sauce, cider vinegar, Dijon mustard, and olive oil. Dress the salad. Add the chickpeas, avocado, onion, garlic, and arugula. Top with sesame seeds.
5. Bon appétit!

105.Herbed Eggplant

Servings:2
Cooking Time:15 Minutes
Ingredients:
- 1 large eggplant, cubed
- ½ teaspoon dried marjoram, crushed
- ½ teaspoon dried oregano, crushed
- ½ teaspoon dried thyme, crushed
- ½ teaspoon garlic powder
- Salt and black pepper, to taste
- Olive oil cooking spray

Directions:
1. Preheat the Air fryer to 390 °F and grease an Air fryer basket.
2. Mix herbs, garlic powder, salt, and black pepper in a bowl.
3. Spray the eggplant cubes with cooking spray and rub with the herb mixture.
4. Arrange the eggplant cubes in the Air fryer basket and cook for about 15 minutes, flipping twice in between.
5. Dish out onto serving plates and serve hot.

106.Jacket Potatoes

Servings:2
Cooking Time: 15 Minutes
Ingredients:
- 2 potatoes
- 1 tablespoon mozzarella cheese, shredded
- 3 tablespoons sour cream
- 1 tablespoon butter, softened
- 1 teaspoon chives, minced
- Salt and ground black pepper, as required

Directions:
1. Set the temperature of air fryer to 355 degrees F. Grease an air fryer basket.
2. With a fork, prick the potatoes.
3. Arrange potatoes into the prepared air fryer basket.
4. Air fry for about 15 minutes.
5. In a bowl, add the remaining ingredients and mix until well combined.
6. Remove from air fryer and transfer the potatoes onto a platter.
7. Open potatoes from the center and stuff them with cheese mixture.
8. Serve immediately

107.Air Fried Halloumi With Veggies

Servings:2
Cooking Time: 15 Minutes
Ingredients:
- 2 zucchinis, cut into even chunks
- 1 large carrot, cut into chunks
- 1 large eggplant, peeled, cut into chunks
- 2 tsp olive oil
- 1 tsp dried mixed herbs
- Salt and black pepper

Directions:

1. In a bowl, add halloumi, zucchini, carrot, eggplant, olive oil, herbs, salt and pepper. Sprinkle with oil, salt and pepper. Arrange halloumi and veggies on the air fryer basket and drizzle with olive oil. Cook for 14 minutes at 340 F, shaking once. Sprinkle with mixed herbs to serve.

108.Italian Seasoned Easy Pasta Chips

Servings:2
Cooking Time:10 Minutes
Ingredients:
- ½ teaspoon salt
- 1 ½ teaspoon Italian seasoning blend
- 1 tablespoon nutritional yeast
- 1 tablespoon olive oil
- 2 cups whole wheat bowtie pasta

Directions:
1. Place the baking dish accessory in the air fryer.
2. Give a good stir.
3. Close the air fryer and cook for 10 minutes at 390 °F.

109.Greek-style Roasted Vegetables

Servings: 3
Cooking Time: 25 Minutes
Ingredients:
- 1/2 pound butternut squash, peeled and cut into 1-inch chunks
- 1/2 pound cauliflower, cut into 1-inch florets
- 1/2 pound zucchini, cut into 1-inch chunks
- 1 red onion, sliced
- 2 bell peppers, cut into 1-inch chunks
- 2 tablespoons extra-virgin olive oil
- 1 cup dry white wine
- 1 teaspoon dried rosemary
- Sea salt and freshly cracked black pepper, to taste

- 1/2 teaspoon dried basil
- 1 (28-ounce) canned diced tomatoes with juice
- 1/2 cup Kalamata olives, pitted

Directions:

1. Toss the vegetables with the olive oil, wine, rosemary, salt, black pepper, and basil until well coated.
2. Pour 1/2 of the canned diced tomatoes into a lightly greased baking dish; spread to cover the bottom of the baking dish.
3. Add the vegetables and top with the remaining diced tomatoes. Scatter the Kalamata olives over the top.
4. Bake in the preheated Air Fryer at 390 degrees F for 20 minutes, rotating the dish halfway through the cooking time. Serve warm and enjoy!

110.Chinese Cabbage Bake

Servings: 4
Cooking Time: 35 Minutes
Ingredients:

- 1/2 pound Chinese cabbage, roughly chopped
- 2 bell peppers, seeded and sliced
- 1 jalapeno pepper, seeded and sliced
- 1 onion, thickly sliced
- 2 garlic cloves, sliced
- 1/2 stick butter
- 4 tablespoons flaxseed meal
- 1/2 cup milk
- 1 cup cream cheese
- Sea salt and freshly ground black pepper, to taste
- 1/2 teaspoon cayenne pepper
- 1 cup Monterey Jack cheese, shredded

Directions:

1. Heat a pan of salted water and bring to a boil. Boil the Chinese cabbage for

2 to 3 minutes. Transfer the Chinese cabbage to cold water to stop the cooking process.
2. Place the Chinese cabbage in a lightly greased casserole dish. Add the peppers, onion, and garlic.
3. Next, melt the butter in a saucepan over a moderate heat. Gradually add the flaxseed meal and cook for 2 minutes to form a paste.
4. Slowly pour in the milk, stirring continuously until a thick sauce forms. Add the cream cheese. Season with the salt, black pepper, and cayenne pepper. Add the mixture to the casserole dish.
5. Top with the shredded Monterey Jack cheese and bake in the preheated Air Fryer at 390 degrees F for 25 minutes. Serve hot.

111.Marinated Tofu Bowl With Pearl Onions

Servings: 4
Cooking Time: 1 Hour 20 Minutes
Ingredients:

- 16 ounces firm tofu, pressed and cut into 1-inch pieces
- 2 tablespoons vegan Worcestershire sauce
- 1 tablespoon apple cider vinegar
- 1 tablespoon maple syrup
- 1/2 teaspoon shallot powder
- 1/2 teaspoon porcini powder
- 1/2 teaspoon garlic powder
- 2 tablespoons peanut oil
- 1 cup pearl onions, peeled

Directions:

1. Place the tofu, Worcestershire sauce, vinegar, maple syrup, shallot powder, porcini powder, and garlic powder in

a ceramic dish. Let it marinate in your refrigerator for 1 hour.

2. Transfer the tofu to the lightly greased Air Fryer basket. Add the peanut oil and pearl onions; toss to combine.
3. Cook the tofu with the pearl onions in the preheated Air Fryer at 380 degrees F for 6 minutes; pause and brush with the reserved marinade; cook for a further 5 minutes.
4. Serve immediately. Bon appétit!

112.Crunchy Eggplant Rounds

Servings: 4
Cooking Time: 45 Minutes
Ingredients:
- 1 (1-pound) eggplant, sliced
- 1/2 cup flax meal
- 1/2 cup rice flour
- Coarse sea salt and ground black pepper, to taste
- 1 teaspoon paprika
- 1 cup water
- 1 cup cornbread crumbs, crushed
- 1/2 cup vegan parmesan

Directions:
1. Toss the eggplant with 1 tablespoon of salt and let it stand for 30 minutes. Drain and rinse well.
2. Mix the flax meal, rice flour, salt, black pepper, and paprika in a bowl. Then, pour in the water and whisk to combine well.
3. In another shallow bowl, mix the cornbread crumbs and vegan parmesan.
4. Dip the eggplant slices in the flour mixture, then in the crumb mixture; press to coat on all sides. Transfer to the lightly greased Air Fryer basket.

5. Cook at 370 degrees F for 6 minutes. Turn each slice over and cook an additional 5 minutes.
6. Serve garnished with spicy ketchup if desired. Bon appétit!

113.Spicy Mixed Veggie Bites

Servings:1
Cooking Time: 30 Minutes
Ingredients:
- 6 medium carrots, diced
- 1 medium broccoli, cut in florets
- 1 onion, diced
- ½ cup garden peas
- 2 leeks, sliced thinly
- 1 small zucchini, chopped
- ⅓ cup flour
- 1 tbsp garlic paste
- 2 tbsp olive oil
- 1 tbsp curry paste
- 2 tsp mixed spice
- 1 tsp coriander
- 1 tsp cumin powder
- 1 ½ cups milk
- 1 tsp ginger paste
- Salt and pepper to taste

Directions:
1. In a pot, steam all vegetables, except the leek and courgette for 10 minutes; set aside. Place a wok over medium heat and add onion, ginger, garlic and olive oil. Stir-fry until onions turn transparent. Add in leek, zucchini and curry paste. Cook for 5 minutes. Add all spices and milk; simmer for 10 minutes.
2. Once the sauce has reduced, add the steamed veggies; mix evenly. Transfer to a bowl and refrigerate for 1 hour. Remove the veggie base from the fridge and mold into bite sizes. Arrange the veggie bites in the fryer

basket and cook at 350 F for 10 minutes. Once ready, serve warm with yogurt sauce.

114. Vegetable Tortilla Pizza

Servings:1
Cooking Time: 15 Minutes
Ingredients:
- ¼ cup grated cheddar cheese
- ¼ cup grated mozzarella cheese
- 1 tbsp cooked sweet corn
- 4 zucchini slices
- 4 eggplant slices
- 4 red onion rings
- ½ green bell pepper, chopped
- 3 cherry tomatoes, quartered
- 1 tortilla
- ¼ tsp basil
- ¼ tsp oregano

Directions:
1. Preheat the air fryer to 350 F. Spread the tomato paste on the tortilla. Arrange the zucchini and eggplant slices first, then green peppers, and onion rings.
2. Arrange the cherry tomatoes and sprinkle the sweet corn over. Sprinkle with oregano and basil and top with cheddar and mozzarella. Place in the fryer and cook for 10 minutes.

115. Herbed Carrots

Servings:8
Cooking Time:14 Minutes
Ingredients:
- 6 large carrots, peeled and sliced lengthwise
- 2 tablespoons olive oil
- ½ tablespoon fresh oregano, chopped
- ½ tablespoon fresh parsley, chopped
- Salt and black pepper, to taste

- 2 tablespoons olive oil, divided
- ½ cup fat-free Italian dressing
- Salt, to taste

Directions:
1. Preheat the Air fryer to 360 °F and grease an Air fryer basket.
2. Mix the carrot slices and olive oil in a bowl and toss to coat well.
3. Arrange the carrot slices in the Air fryer basket and cook for about 12 minutes.
4. Dish out the carrot slices onto serving plates and sprinkle with herbs, salt and black pepper.
5. Transfer into the Air fryer basket and cook for 2 more minutes.
6. Dish out and serve hot.

116. Spaghetti Squash

Servings: 2
Cooking Time: 45 Minutes
Ingredients:
- spaghetti squash
- 1 tsp. olive oil
- Salt and pepper
- 4 tbsp. heavy cream
- 1 tsp. butter

Directions:
1. Pre-heat your fryer at 360°F.
2. Cut and de-seed the spaghetti squash. Brush with the olive oil and season with salt and pepper to taste.
3. Put the squash inside the fryer, placing it cut-side-down. Cook for thirty minutes. Halfway through cooking, fluff the spaghetti inside the squash with a fork.
4. When the squash is ready, fluff the spaghetti some more, then pour some heavy cream and butter over it and give it a good stir. Serve with the low-carb tomato sauce of your choice.

117.Butternut Squash Chili

Servings: 4
Cooking Time: 35 Minutes
Ingredients:
- 2 tablespoons canola oil
- 1 cup leeks, chopped
- 2 garlic cloves, crushed
- 2 ripe tomatoes, pureed
- 2 chipotle peppers in adobo, chopped
- 1 teaspoon ground cumin
- 1 teaspoon chili powder
- Kosher salt and ground black pepper, to your liking
- 1 cup vegetable broth
- 1 pound butternut squash, peeled and diced into 1/2-inch chunks
- 16 ounces canned kidney beans, drained and rinsed
- 1 avocado, pitted, peeled and diced

Directions:
1. Start by preheating your Air Fryer to 365 degrees F.
2. Heat the oil in a baking pan until sizzling. Then, sauté the leeks and garlic in the baking pan. Cook for 4 to 6 minutes.
3. Now, add the tomatoes, chipotle peppers, cumin, chili powder, salt, pepper, and vegetable broth. Cook for 15 minutes, stirring every 5 minutes.
4. Stir in the the butternut squash and canned beans; let it cook for a further 8 minutes, stirring halfway through the cooking time.
5. Serve in individual bowls, garnished with the avocado. Enjoy!

118.Ooey-gooey Dessert Quesadilla

Servings: 2
Cooking Time: 25 Minutes
Ingredients:
- 1/4 cup blueberries
- 1/4 cup fresh orange juice
- 1/2 tablespoon maple syrup
- 1/2 cup vegan cream cheese
- 1 teaspoon vanilla extract
- 2 (6-inch tortillas
- 2 teaspoons coconut oil
- 1/4 cup vegan dark chocolate

Directions:
1. Bring the blueberries, orange juice, and maple syrup to a boil in a saucepan. Reduce the heat and let it simmer until the sauce thickens, about 10 minutes.
2. In a mixing dish, combine the cream cheese with the vanilla extract; spread on the tortillas. Add the blueberry filling on top. Fold in half.
3. Place the quesadillas in the greased Air Fryer basket. Cook at 390 degrees F for 10 minutes, until tortillas are golden brown and filling is melted. Make sure to turn them over halfway through the cooking.
4. Heat the coconut oil in a small pan and add the chocolate; whisk to combine well. Drizzle the chocolate sauce over the quesadilla and serve. Enjoy!

119.Your Traditional Mac 'n Cheese

Servings:3
Cooking Time: 32 Minutes
Ingredients:
- 1/2 pinch ground nutmeg
- 1/2 teaspoon Dijon mustard
- 1/2 teaspoon salt
- 1/4 cup panko bread crumbs
- 1/8 teaspoon cayenne pepper
- 1/8 teaspoon dried thyme
- 1/8 teaspoon white pepper
- 1/8 teaspoon Worcestershire sauce
- 1-1/2 cups milk

- 1-1/2 cups shredded sharp Cheddar cheese, divided
- 1-1/2 teaspoons butter, melted
- 2 tablespoons all-purpose flour
- 2 tablespoons butter
- 8-ounce elbow macaroni, cooked according to package Directions:

Directions:
1. Melt 2 tbsp butter in baking pan of air fryer for 2 minutes at 360°F. Stir in flour and cook for 3 minutes, stirring every now and then. Stir in white pepper, cayenne pepper, and thyme. Cook for 2 minutes. Stir in a cup of milk and whisk well. Cook for 5 minutes while mixing constantly.
2. Mix in salt, Worcestershire sauce, and nutmeg . Mix well. Cook for 5 minutes or until thickened while stirring frequently.
3. Add cheese and mix well. Cook for 3 minutes or until melted and thoroughly mixed.
4. Stir in Dijon mustard and mix well. Add macaroni and toss well to coat. Sprinkle remaining cheese on top.
5. In a small bowl mix well 1 ½ tsp butter and panko. Sprinkle on top of cheese.
6. Cook for 15 minutes at 390°F until tops are lightly browned.
7. Serve and enjoy.

120.Roasted Chat-masala Spiced Broccoli

Servings:2
Cooking Time:15 Minutes
Ingredients:
- ¼ teaspoon chat masala
- ¼ teaspoons turmeric powder
- ½ teaspoon salt
- 1 tablespoon chickpea flour
- 2 cups broccoli florets

- 2 tablespoons yogurt

Directions:
1. Place all ingredients in a bowl and toss the broccoli florets to combine.
2. Place the baking dish accessory in the air fryer and place the broccoli florets.
3. Close the air fryer and cook for 15 minutes at 330 °F.
4. Halfway through the cooking time, give the baking dish a shake.

121.Cottage Cheese And Potatoes

Servings:5
Cooking Time: 30 Minutes
Ingredients:
- 1 bunch asparagus, trimmed
- ¼ cup fresh cream
- ¼ cup cottage cheese, cubed
- 1 tbsp whole-grain mustard

Directions:
1. Preheat the air fryer to 400 F and place the potatoes in the basket; cook for 25 minutes. Boil salted water in a pot over medium heat. Add asparagus and cook for 3 minutes until tender.
2. In a bowl, mix cooked potatoes, cottage cheese, cream, asparagus and mustard. Toss well and season with salt and black pepper. Transfer the mixture to the potato skin shells and serve.

122.Delightful Mushrooms

Servings:4
Cooking Time:22 Minutes
Ingredients:
- 2 cups mushrooms, sliced
- 2 tablespoons cheddar cheese, shredded
- 1 tablespoon fresh chives, chopped
- 2 tablespoons olive oil

Directions:

1. Preheat the Air fryer to 355 °F and grease an Air fryer basket.
2. Coat the mushrooms with olive oil and arrange into the Air fryer basket.
3. Cook for about 20 minutes and dish out in a platter.
4. Top with chives and cheddar cheese and cook for 2 more minutes.
5. Dish out and serve warm.

123.Paneer Cutlet

Servings:1
Cooking Time: 15 Minutes
Ingredients:
- 1 cup grated cheese
- ½ tsp chai masala
- 1 tsp butter
- ½ tsp garlic powder
- 1 small onion, finely chopped
- ½ tsp oregano
- ½ tsp salt

Directions:
1. Preheat the air fryer to 350 F, and grease a baking dish. Mix all ingredients in a bowl, until well incorporated. Make cutlets out of the mixture and place them on the greased baking dish. Place the baking dish in the air fryer and cook the cutlets for 10 minutes, until crispy.

124.Paneer Cheese Balls

Servings:2
Cooking Time: 12 Minutes
Ingredients:
- 2 tbsp flour
- 2 medium onions, chopped
- 1 tbsp cornflour
- 1 green chili, chopped
- 1-inch ginger piece, chopped
- 1 tsp red chili powder
- A few leaves of coriander, chopped
- oil and salt

Directions:
1. Mix all ingredients, except the oil and cheese. Take a small part of the mixture, roll it up and slowly press it to flatten. Stuff in 1 cube of cheese and seal the edges. Repeat with the rest of the mixture. Fry the balls in the fryer for 12 minutes and at 370 F. Serve hot with ketchup!

POULTRY RECIPES

125. Quick And Crispy Chicken

Servings: 4
Cooking Time: 15 Minutes
Ingredients:
- 2 tbsp butter
- 2 oz breadcrumbs
- 1 large egg, whisked

Directions:
1. Preheat air fryer to 380 F. Combine butter the breadcrumbs in a bowl. Keep mixing and stirring until the mixture gets crumbly. Dip the chicken in the egg wash. Then dip the chicken in the crumbs mix. Cook for 10 minutes. Serve.

126. Buttery Chicken Wings

Servings: 4
Cooking Time: 30 Minutes
Ingredients:
- 2 pounds chicken wings
- Salt and black pepper to the taste
- 3 garlic cloves, minced
- 3 tablespoons butter, melted
- ½ cup heavy cream
- ½ teaspoon basil, dried
- ½ teaspoon oregano, dried
- ¼ cup parmesan, grated

Directions:
1. In a baking dish that fits your air fryer, mix the chicken wings with all the ingredients except the parmesan and toss. Put the dish to your air fryer and cook at 380 degrees F for 30 minutes. Sprinkle the cheese on top, leave the mix aside for 10 minutes, divide between plates and serve.

127. Tomato, Eggplant 'n Chicken Skewers

Servings: 4
Cooking Time: 25 Minutes
Ingredients:
- ¼ teaspoon cayenne pepper
- ¼ teaspoon ground cardamom
- 1 ½ teaspoon ground turmeric
- 1 can coconut milk
- 1 cup cherry tomatoes
- 1 medium eggplant, cut into cubes
- 1 onion, cut into wedges
- 1-inch ginger, grated
- 2 pounds boneless chicken breasts, cut into cubes
- 2 tablespoons fresh lime juice
- 2 tablespoons tomato paste
- 3 teaspoons lime zest
- 4 cloves of garlic, minced
- Salt and pepper to taste

Directions:
1. Place in a bowl the garlic, ginger, coconut milk, lime zest, lime juice, tomato paste, salt, pepper, turmeric, cayenne pepper, cardamom, and chicken breasts. Allow to marinate in the fridge for at least for 2 hours.
2. Preheat the air fryer to 390 °F.
3. Place the grill pan accessory in the air fryer.
4. Skewer the chicken cubes with eggplant, onion, and cherry tomatoes on bamboo skewers.
5. Place on the grill pan and cook for 25 minutes making sure to flip the chicken every 5 minutes for even cooking.

128. Coriander Chicken Breast

Servings: 5
Cooking Time: 20 Minutes
Ingredients:

- 15 oz chicken breast, skinless, boneless
- 1 teaspoon lemongrass
- 1 teaspoon ground black pepper
- 1 teaspoon salt
- 1 teaspoon chili powder
- 1 teaspoon smoked paprika
- 2 teaspoons apple cider vinegar
- 1 teaspoon lemon juice
- 1 tablespoon sunflower oil
- 1 teaspoon dried basil
- ½ teaspoon ground coriander
- 2 tablespoons water
- 1 tablespoon heavy cream

Directions:

1. Make the marinade: In the bowl mix up lemongrass, ground black pepper, salt, chili powder, smoked paprika, apple cider vinegar, lemon juice, sunflower oil, dried basil, ground coriander, water, and heavy cream. Then chop the chicken breast roughly and put it in the marinade. Stir it well and leave for 20 minutes in the fridge. Then preheat the air fryer to 375F. Put the marinated chicken breast pieces in the air fryer and cook them for 20 minutes. Shake the chicken pieces after 10 minutes of cooking to avoid burning. The cooked chicken breast pieces should have a light brown color.

129.Caesar Marinated Grilled Chicken

Servings:3
Cooking Time: 24 Minutes
Ingredients:

- ¼ cup crouton
- 1 teaspoon lemon zest. Form into ovals, skewer and grill.
- 1/2 cup Parmesan
- 1/4 cup breadcrumbs

- 1-pound ground chicken
- 2 tablespoons Caesar dressing and more for drizzling
- 2-4 romaine leaves

Directions:

1. In a shallow dish, mix well chicken, 2 tablespoons Caesar dressing, parmesan, and breadcrumbs. Mix well with hands. Form into 1-inch oval patties.
2. Thread chicken pieces in skewers. Place on skewer rack in air fryer.
3. For 12 minutes, cook on 360°F. Halfway through cooking time, turnover skewers. If needed, cook in batches.
4. Serve and enjoy on a bed of lettuce and sprinkle with croutons and extra dressing.

130.Chicken Popcorn

Servings: 6
Cooking Time: 10 Minutes
Ingredients:

- 4 eggs
- 1 1/2 lbs chicken breasts, cut into small chunks
- 1 tsp paprika
- 1/2 tsp garlic powder
- 1 tsp onion powder
- 2 1/2 cups pork rind, crushed
- 1/4 cup coconut flour
- Pepper
- Salt

Directions:

1. In a small bowl, mix together coconut flour, pepper, and salt.
2. In another bowl, whisk eggs until combined.
3. Take one more bowl and mix together pork panko, paprika, garlic powder, and onion powder.

4. Add chicken pieces in a large mixing bowl. Sprinkle coconut flour mixture over chicken and toss well.
5. Dip chicken pieces in the egg mixture and coat with pork panko mixture and place on a plate.
6. Spray air fryer basket with cooking spray.
7. Preheat the air fryer to 400 F.
8. Add half prepared chicken in air fryer basket and cook for 10-12 minutes. Shake basket halfway through.
9. Cook remaining half using the same method.
10. Serve and enjoy.

131.Chicken & Honey Sauce

Servings: 4
Cooking Time: 20 Minutes
Ingredients:
- 4 chicken sausages
- 2 tbsp. honey
- ¼ cup mayonnaise
- 2 tbsp. Dijon mustard
- 1 tbsp. balsamic vinegar
- ½ tsp. dried rosemary

Directions:
1. Pre-heat your Air Fryer at 350°F.
2. Place the sausages on the grill pan of your fryer and grill for about 13 minutes, flipping them halfway through the cooking time.
3. In the meantime, make the sauce by whisking together the rest of the ingredients.
4. Pour the sauce over the warm sausages before serving.

132.Delicious Turkey Sandwiches

Servings: 4
Cooking Time: 45 Minutes
Ingredients:
- 1 pound turkey tenderloins

- 1 tablespoon Dijon-style mustard
- 1 tablespoon olive oil
- Sea salt and ground black pepper, to taste
- 1 teaspoon Italian seasoning mix
- 1/4 cup all-purpose flour
- 1 cup turkey stock
- 8 slices sourdough, toasted
- 4 tablespoons tomato ketchup
- 4 tablespoons mayonnaise
- 4 pickles, sliced

Directions:
1. Rub the turkey tenderloins with the mustard and olive oil. Season with salt, black pepper, and Italian seasoning mix.
2. Cook the turkey tenderloins at 350 degrees F for 30 minutes, flipping them over halfway through. Let them rest for 5 to 7 minutes before slicing.
3. For the gravy, in a saucepan, place the drippings from the roasted turkey. Add 1/8 cup of flour and 1/2 cup of turkey stock; whisk until it makes a smooth paste.
4. Once it gets a golden brown color, add the rest of the stock and flour. Season with salt to taste. Let it simmer over medium heat, stirring constantly for 6 to 7 minutes.
5. Assemble the sandwiches with the turkey, gravy, tomato ketchup, mayonnaise, and pickles. Serve and enjoy!

133.Marrod's Meatballs

Servings: 6
Cooking Time: 15 Minutes
Ingredients:
- 1 lb. ground turkey
- 1 tbsp. fresh mint leaves, finely chopped

- 1 tsp. onion powder
- 1 ½ teaspoons garlic paste
- 1 tsp. crushed red pepper flakes
- ¼ cup melted butter
- ¾ tsp. fine sea salt
- ¼ cup grated Pecorino Romano

Directions:
1. In a bowl, combine all of the ingredients well. Using an ice cream scoop, mold the meat into balls.
2. Air fry the meatballs at 380°F for about 7 minutes, in batches if necessary. Shake the basket frequently throughout the cooking time for even results.
3. Serve with basil leaves and tomato sauce if desired.

134.Crispy Chicken Tenders With Hot Aioli

Servings:4
Cooking Time: 15 Minutes
Ingredients:
- 4 tbsp olive oil
- 1 cup breadcrumbs
- Salt and pepper to taste
- ½ tbsp garlic powder
- ½ tbsp ground chili
- Aioli:
- ½ cup mayonnaise
- 2 tbsp olive oil
- ½ tbsp ground chili

Directions:
1. Mix breadcrumbs, salt, pepper, garlic powder and chili, and spread onto a plate. Spray the chicken with oil. Roll the strips in the breadcrumb mixture until well coated. Spray with a little bit of oil.
2. Arrange an even layer of strips into your air fryer and cook for 6 minutes at 360 F, turning once halfway

through. To prepare the hot aioli: combine mayo with oil and ground chili. Serve hot.

135.Lemon-parsley Chicken Packets

Servings:4
Cooking Time: 45 Minutes
Ingredients:
- ¼ cup smoked paprika
- ½ cup parsley leaves
- ½ teaspoon liquid smoke seasoning
- 1 ½ tablespoon cayenne pepper
- 2 pounds chicken thighs
- 4 lemons, halved
- Salt and pepper to taste

Directions:
1. Preheat the air fryer to 390 °F.
2. Place the grill pan accessory in the air fryer.
3. In a large foil, place the chicken and season with paprika, liquid smoke seasoning, salt, pepper, and cayenne pepper.
4. Top with lemon and parsley.
5. Place on the grill and cook for 45 minutes.

136.Cayenne And Turmeric Chicken Strips

Servings: 6
Cooking Time: 14 Minutes
Ingredients:
- 2-pound chicken breast, skinless, boneless
- 1 teaspoon salt
- 1 teaspoon ground turmeric
- ½ teaspoon cayenne pepper
- 1 egg, beaten
- 2 tablespoons coconut flour

Directions:
1. Cut the chicken breast into the strips and sprinkle with salt, ground turmeric, and cayenne pepper. Then

add beaten egg in the chicken strips and stir the mixture. After this, add coconut flour and stir it. Preheat the air fryer to 400F. Put ½ part of all chicken strips in the air fryer basket in one layer and cook them for 7 minutes. Repeat the same steps with the remaining chicken strips.

137.Lebanese Style Grilled Chicken

Servings:3
Cooking Time: 20 Minutes
Ingredients:

- 1 onion, cut into large chunks
- 1 small green bell pepper, cut into large chunks
- 1 teaspoon tomato paste
- 1/2 cup chopped fresh flat-leaf parsley
- 1/2 teaspoon dried oregano
- 1/3 cup plain yogurt
- 1/8 teaspoon ground allspice
- 1/8 teaspoon ground black pepper
- 1/8 teaspoon ground cardamom
- 1/8 teaspoon ground cinnamon
- 1-pound skinless, boneless chicken breast halves cut into 2-inch pieces
- 2 cloves garlic, minced
- 2 tablespoons lemon juice
- 2 tablespoons vegetable oil
- 3/4 teaspoon salt

Directions:

1. In a resealable plastic bag, mix cardamom, cinnamon, allspice, pepper, oregano, salt, tomato paste, garlic, yogurt, vegetable oil, and lemon juice. Add chicken, remove excess air, seal, and marinate in the ref for at least 4 hours.
2. Thread chicken into skewers, place on skewer rack and cook in batches.

3. For 10 minutes, cook on 360°F. Halfway through cooking time, turnover skewers.
4. Serve and enjoy with a sprinkle of parsley.

138.Spicy Peach Glazed Grilled Chicken

Servings:4
Cooking Time: 40 Minutes
Ingredients:

- 2 cups peach preserves
- 2 pounds chicken thighs
- 3 tablespoons olive oil
- 2 tablespoons soy sauce
- 1 tablespoons Dijon mustard
- 1 tablespoon chili powder
- 1 tablespoon minced garlic
- 1 jalapeno chopped
- Salt and pepper to taste

Directions:

1. Place all ingredients in a Ziploc bag and allow to rest in the fridge for at least 2 hours.
2. Preheat the air fryer at 375 °F.
3. Place the grill pan accessory in the air fryer.
4. Grill for 40 minutes while flipping the chicken every 10 minutes.
5. Meanwhile, pour the marinade in a saucepan and allow to simmer for 5 minutes until the sauce thickens.
6. Brush the chicken with the glaze before serving.

139.Chicken Thighs Recipe

Servings: 6
Cooking Time:30 Minutes
Ingredients:

- 2 ½ lbs. chicken thighs
- 5 green onions; chopped
- 2 tbsp. sesame oil
- 1 tbsp. sherry wine

- 1/2 tsp. white vinegar
- 1 tbsp. soy sauce
- 1/4 tsp. sugar
- Salt and black pepper to the taste

Directions:
1. Season chicken with salt and pepper, rub with half of the sesame oil, add to your air fryer and cook at 360 °F, for 20 minutes.
2. Meanwhile; heat up a pan with the rest of the oil over medium high heat, add green onions, sherry wine, vinegar, soy sauce and sugar; toss, cover and cook for 10 minutes. Shred chicken using 2 forks divide among plates, drizzle sauce all over and serve.

140.Randy's Roasted Chicken

Servings: 4
Cooking Time: 55 Minutes
Ingredients:
- 5 – 7 lb. whole chicken with skin
- 1 tsp. garlic powder
- 1 tsp. onion powder
- ½ tsp. dried thyme
- ½ tsp. dried basil
- ½ tsp. dried rosemary
- ½ tsp. black pepper
- 2 tsp. salt
- 2 tbsp. extra virgin olive oil

Directions:
1. Massage the salt, pepper, herbs, and olive oil into the chicken. Allow to marinade for a minimum of 20 – 30 minutes.
2. In the meantime, pre-heat the Air Fryer to 340 F.
3. Place the chicken in the fryer and cook for 18 – 20 minutes.
4. Flip the chicken over and cook for an additional 20 minutes.

5. Leave the chicken to rest for about 10 minutes before carving and serving.

141.Smoked Duck With Rosemary-infused Gravy

Servings: 4
Cooking Time: 30 Minutes
Ingredients:
- 1 ½ pounds smoked duck breasts, boneless
- 1 tablespoon yellow mustard
- 2 tablespoons ketchup
- 1 teaspoon agave syrup
- 12 pearl onions peeled
- 1 tablespoon flour
- 5 ounces chicken broth
- 1 teaspoon rosemary, finely chopped

Directions:
1. Cook the smoked duck breasts in the preheated Air Fryer at 365 degrees F for 15 minutes.
2. Smear the mustard, ketchup, and agave syrup on the duck breast. Top with pearl onions. Cook for a further 7 minutes or until the skin of the duck breast looks crispy and golden brown.
3. Slice the duck breasts and reserve. Drain off the duck fat from the pan.
4. Then, add the reserved 1 tablespoon of duck fat to the pan and warm it over medium heat; add flour and cook until your roux is dark brown.
5. Add the chicken broth and rosemary to the pan. Reduce the heat to low and cook until the gravy has thickened slightly. Spoon the warm gravy over the reserved duck breasts. Enjoy!

142.Spicy Turkey Patties With Chive Mayonnaise

Servings: 6

Cooking Time: 20 Minutes

Ingredients:

- For the Turkey Sliders:
- 3/4 pound turkey mince
- 1/4 cup pickled jalapeno, chopped
- 1 tablespoon oyster sauce
- 1-2 cloves garlic, minced
- 1 tablespoon chopped fresh cilantro
- 2 tablespoons chopped scallions
- Sea salt and ground black pepper, to savor
- For the Chive Mayo:
- 1 cup mayonnaise
- 1 tablespoon chives
- 1 teaspoon salt
- Zest of 1 lime

Directions:

1. In a mixing bowl, thoroughly combine all ingredients for the turkey patties.
2. Mold the mixture into 6 even-sized slider patties. Then, air-fry them at 365 degrees F for 15 minutes.
3. Meanwhile, make the Chive Mayonnaise by mixing the rest of the above ingredients. Serve warm.

143.Sweet And Sour Chicken Thighs

Servings:2
Cooking Time:20 Minutes

Ingredients:

- 1 scallion, finely chopped
- 2 (4-ounces) skinless, boneless chicken thighs
- ½ cup corn flour
- 1 garlic clove, minced
- ½ tablespoon soy sauce
- ½ tablespoon rice vinegar
- 1 teaspoon sugar
- Salt and black pepper, as required

Directions:

1. Preheat the Air fryer to 390 °F and grease an Air fryer basket.

2. Mix all the ingredients except chicken and corn flour in a bowl.
3. Place the corn flour in another bowl.
4. Coat the chicken thighs into the marinade and then dredge into the corn flour.
5. Arrange the chicken thighs into the Air Fryer basket, skin side down and cook for about 10 minutes.
6. Set the Air fryer to 355 °F and cook for 10 more minutes.
7. Dish out the chicken thighs onto a serving platter and serve hot.

144.Fried Chicken Halves

Servings: 4
Cooking Time: 75 Minutes

Ingredients:

- 16 oz whole chicken
- 1 tablespoon dried thyme
- 1 teaspoon ground cumin
- 1 teaspoon salt
- 1 tablespoon avocado oil

Directions:

1. Cut the chicken into halves and sprinkle it with dried thyme, cumin, and salt. Then brush the chicken halves with avocado oil. Preheat the air fryer to 365F. Put the chicken halves in the air fryer and cook them for 60 minutes. Then flip the chicken halves on another side and cook them for 15 minutes more.

145.Teriyaki Chicken

Servings: 2
Cooking Time: 30 Minutes

Ingredients:

- 2 boneless chicken drumsticks
- 1 tsp. ginger, grated
- 1 tbsp. cooking wine
- 3 tbsp. teriyaki sauce

Directions:

1. Combine all of the ingredients in a bowl. Refrigerate for half an hour.
2. Place the chicken in the Air Fryer baking pan and fry at 350°F for 8 minutes. Turn the chicken over and raise the temperature to 380°F. Allow to cook for another 6 minutes. Serve hot.

146.Crispy 'n Salted Chicken Meatballs

Servings:6
Cooking Time: 20 Minutes
Ingredients:

- ½ cup almond flour
- ¾ pound skinless boneless chicken breasts, ground
- 1 ½ teaspoon herbs de Provence
- 1 tablespoon coconut milk
- 2 eggs, beaten
- Salt and pepper to taste

Directions:

1. Mix all ingredient in a bowl.
2. Form small balls using the palms of your hands.
3. Place in the fridge to set for at least 2 hours.
4. Preheat the air fryer for 5 minutes.
5. Place the chicken balls in the fryer basket.
6. Cook for 20 minutes at 325 °F.
7. Halfway through the cooking time, give the fryer basket a shake to cook evenly on all sides.

147.Crispy Chicken Thighs

Servings: 1
Cooking Time: 35 Minutes
Ingredients:

- 1 lb. chicken thighs
- Salt and pepper
- 2 cups roasted pecans

- 1 cup water
- 1 cup flour

Directions:

1. Pre-heat your fryer to 400°F.
2. Season the chicken with salt and pepper, then set aside.
3. Pulse the roasted pecans in a food processor until a flour-like consistency is achieved.
4. Fill a dish with the water, another with the flour, and a third with the pecans.
5. Coat the thighs with the flour. Mix the remaining flour with the processed pecans.
6. Dredge the thighs in the water and then press into the -pecan mix, ensuring the chicken is completely covered.
7. Cook the chicken in the fryer for twenty-two minutes, with an extra five minutes added if you would like the chicken a darker-brown color. Check the temperature has reached 165°F before serving.

148.Country-fried Chicken Drumsticks

Servings:4
Cooking Time: 20 Minutes
Ingredients:

- 1 tsp garlic powder
- 1 tsp cayenne pepper
- ½ cup flour
- ¼ cup milk
- ¼ tbsp lemon juice
- Salt and black pepper to taste

Directions:

1. Preheat your Air Fryer to 390 F. Spray the air fryer basket with cooking spray.
2. In a small bowl, mix garlic powder, cayenne pepper, salt, and black

pepper. Rub the chicken drumsticks with the mixture. In a separate bowl, combine milk with lemon juice. Pour the flour on a plate.

3. Dunk the chicken in the milk mixture, then roll in the flour to coat
4. Place the chicken in the cooking basket and spray it with cooking spray. Cook for 6 minutes, Slide out the fryer basket and flip; cook for 6 more minutes. Serve cooled.

149.Creamy Duck Strips

Servings: 5
Cooking Time: 17 Minutes
Ingredients:
- 12 oz duck breast, skinless, boneless
- ½ cup coconut flour
- 1/3 cup heavy cream
- 1 teaspoon salt
- 1 teaspoon white pepper

Directions:
1. Cut the duck breast on the small strips (fingers) and sprinkle with salt and white pepper. Then dip the duck fingers in the heavy cream and coat in the coconut flour. Preheat the air fryer to 375F. Put the duck fingers in the air fryer basket in one layer and cook them for 10 minutes. Then flip the duck fingers on another side and cook them for 7 minutes more.

150.Crusted Chicken

Servings: 2
Cooking Time: 30 Minutes
Ingredients:
- ¼ cup slivered s
- 2x 6-oz. boneless skinless chicken breasts
- 2 tbsp. full-fat mayonnaise
- 1 tbsp. Dijon mustard

Directions:
1. Pulse the s in a food processor until they are finely chopped. Spread the s on a plate and set aside.
2. Cut each chicken breast in half lengthwise.
3. Mix the mayonnaise and mustard together and then spread evenly on top of the chicken slices.
4. Place the chicken into the plate of chopped s to coat completely, laying each coated slice into the basket of your fryer.
5. Cook for 25 minutes at 350°F until golden. Test the temperature, making sure the chicken has reached 165°F. Serve hot.

151.Finger-lickin' Vermouth And Honey Turkey

Servings:4
Cooking Time:55 Minutes + Marinating Time
Ingredients:
- 1 teaspoon marjoram
- 1 teaspoon dried oregano
- 1 tablespoon honey
- 1/4 cup vermouth
- 2 tablespoons lemon juice
- 1 turkey tenderloin, quartered
- 1 tablespoon sesame oil
- Sea salt flakes, to savor
- 1/2 teaspoon freshly ground pepper, or to savor
- 3/4 teaspoon smoked paprika
- 1 teaspoon crushed sage leaves, dried

Directions:
1. Place the first 6 ingredients in a mixing dish; let it marinate for 3 hours at least.
2. Then, drizzle the turkey breasts with sesame oil and add the other ingredients.

3. Lastly, roast in the Air Fryer cooking basket about 50 to 55 minutes at 355 degrees F; make sure to turn them over a few times during the cooking time.

152.Baked Rice, Black Bean And Cheese

Servings:4
Cooking Time: 62 Minutes
Ingredients:
- 1 cooked skinless boneless chicken breast halves, chopped
- 1 cup shredded Swiss cheese
- 1/2 (15 ounce) can black beans, drained
- 1/2 (4 ounce) can diced green chile peppers, drained
- 1/2 cup vegetable broth
- 1/2 medium zucchini, thinly sliced
- 1/4 cup sliced mushrooms
- 1/4 teaspoon cumin
- 1-1/2 teaspoons olive oil
- 2 tablespoons and 2 teaspoons diced onion
- 3 tablespoons brown rice
- 3 tablespoons shredded carrots
- ground cayenne pepper to taste
- salt to taste

Directions:
1. Lightly grease baking pan of air fryer with cooking spray. Add rice and broth. Cover pan with foil cook for 10 minutes at 390°F. Lower heat to 300°F and fluff rice. Cook for another 10 minutes. Let it stand for 10 minutes and transfer to a bowl and set aside.
2. Add oil to same baking pan. Stir in onion and cook for 5 minutes at 330°F.

3. Stir in mushrooms, chicken, and zucchini. Mix well and cook for 5 minutes.
4. Stir in cayenne pepper, salt, and cumin. Mix well and cook for another 2 minutes.
5. Stir in ½ of the Swiss cheese, carrots, chiles, beans, and rice. Toss well to mix. Evenly spread in pan. Top with remaining cheese.
6. Cover pan with foil.
7. Cook for 15 minutes at 390°F and then remove foil and cook for another 5 to 10 minutes or until tops are lightly browned.
8. Serve and enjoy.

153.Beastly Bbq Drumsticks

Servings: 4
Cooking Time: 45 Minutes
Ingredients:
- 4 chicken drumsticks
- ½ tbsp. mustard
- 1 clove garlic, crushed
- 1 tsp. chili powder
- 2 tsp. sugar
- 1 tbsp. olive oil
- Freshly ground black pepper

Directions:
1. Pre-heat the Air Fryer to 390°F.
2. Mix together the garlic, sugar, mustard, a pinch of salt, freshly ground pepper, chili powder and oil.
3. Massage this mixture into the drumsticks and leave to marinate for a minimum of 20 minutes.
4. Put the drumsticks in the fryer basket and cook for 10 minutes.
5. Bring the temperature down to 300°F and continue to cook the drumsticks for a further10 minutes. When

cooked through, serve with bread and corn salad.

154.Strawberry Turkey

Servings: 2
Cooking Time: 50 Minutes
Ingredients:
- 2 lb. turkey breast
- 1 tbsp. olive oil
- Salt and pepper
- 1 cup fresh strawberries

Directions:
1. Pre-heat your fryer to 375°F.
2. Massage the turkey breast with olive oil, before seasoning with a generous amount of salt and pepper.
3. Cook the turkey in the fryer for fifteen minutes. Flip the turkey and cook for a further fifteen minutes.
4. During these last fifteen minutes, blend the strawberries in a food processor until a smooth consistency has been achieved.
5. Heap the strawberries over the turkey, then cook for a final seven minutes and enjoy.

155.Country-style Nutty Turkey Breast

Servings: 2

Cooking Time: 30 Minutes
Ingredients:
- 1 ½ tablespoons coconut aminos
- 1/2 tablespoon xanthan gum
- 2 bay leaves
- 1/3 cup dry sherry
- 1 ½ tablespoons chopped walnuts
- 1 teaspoon shallot powder
- 1 pound turkey breasts, sliced
- 1 teaspoon garlic powder
- 2 teaspoons olive oil
- 1/2 teaspoon onion salt
- 1/2 teaspoon red pepper flakes, crushed
- 1 teaspoon ground black pepper

Directions:
1. Begin by preheating your Air Fryer to 395 degrees F. Place all ingredients, minus chopped walnuts, in a mixing bowl and let them marinate at least 1 hour.
2. After that, cook the marinated turkey breast approximately 23 minutes or until heated through.
3. Pause the machine, scatter chopped walnuts over the top and air-fry an additional 5 minutes. Bon appétit!

BEEF,PORK & LAMB RECIPES

156.Crispy Roast Garlic-salt Pork

Servings:4
Cooking Time: 45 Minutes
Ingredients:

- 1 teaspoon Chinese five spice powder
- 1 teaspoon white pepper
- 2 pounds pork belly
- 2 teaspoons garlic salt

Directions:

1. Preheat the air fryer to 390 °F.
2. Mix all the spices in a bowl to create the dry rub.
3. Score the skin of the pork belly with a knife and season the entire pork with the spice rub.
4. Place in the air fryer basket and cook for 40 to 45 minutes until the skin is crispy.
5. Chop before serving.

157.Spiced Lamb Steaks

Servings:3
Cooking Time:15 Minutes
Ingredients:

- ½ onion, roughly chopped
- 1½ pounds boneless lamb sirloin steaks
- 5 garlic cloves, peeled
- 1 tablespoon fresh ginger, peeled
- 1 teaspoon garam masala
- 1 teaspoon ground fennel
- ½ teaspoon ground cumin
- ½ teaspoon ground cinnamon
- ½ teaspoon cayenne pepper
- Salt and black pepper, to taste

Directions:

1. Preheat the Air fryer to 330 °F and grease an Air fryer basket.
2. Put the onion, garlic, ginger, and spices in a blender and pulse until smooth.
3. Coat the lamb steaks with this mixture on both sides and refrigerate to marinate for about 24 hours.
4. Arrange the lamb steaks in the Air fryer basket and cook for about 15 minutes, flipping once in between.
5. Dish out the steaks in a platter and serve warm.

158.Moist Stuffed Pork Roll

Servings:4
Cooking Time:15 Minutes
Ingredients:

- 1 scallion, chopped
- ¼ cup sun-dried tomatoes, chopped finely
- 2 tablespoons fresh parsley, chopped
- 4 (6-ounce) pork cutlets, pounded slightly
- Salt and black pepper, to taste
- 2 teaspoons paprika
- ½ tablespoon olive oil

Directions:

1. Preheat the Air fryer to 390 °F and grease an Air fryer basket.
2. Mix scallion, tomatoes, parsley, salt and black pepper in a large bowl.
3. Coat the cutlets with tomato mixture and roll each cutlet.
4. Secure the cutlets with cocktail sticks and rub with paprika, salt and black pepper.
5. Coat evenly with oil and transfer into the Air fryer basket.
6. Cook for about 15 minutes, flipping once in between and dish out to serve hot.

159. Vegetables & Beef Cubes

Servings: 4
Cooking Time: 20 Minutes + Marinating Time
Ingredients:

- 1 lb. top round steak, cut into cubes
- 2 tbsp. olive oil
- 1 tbsp. apple cider vinegar
- 1 tsp. fine sea salt
- ½ tsp. ground black pepper
- 1 tsp. shallot powder
- ¾ tsp. smoked cayenne pepper
- ½ tsp. garlic powder
- ¼ tsp. ground cumin
- ¼ lb. broccoli, cut into florets
- ¼ lb. mushrooms, sliced
- 1 tsp. dried basil
- 1 tsp. celery seeds

Directions:

1. Massage the olive oil, vinegar, salt, black pepper, shallot powder, cayenne pepper, garlic powder, and cumin into the cubed steak, ensuring to coat each piece evenly.
2. Allow to marinate for a minimum of 3 hours.
3. Put the beef cubes in the Air Fryer cooking basket and allow to cook at 365°F for 12 minutes.
4. When the steak is cooked through, place it in a bowl.
5. Wipe the grease from the cooking basket and pour in the vegetables. Season them with basil and celery seeds.
6. Cook at 400°F for 5 to 6 minutes. When the vegetables are hot, serve them with the steak.

160. Cornbread, Ham 'n Eggs Frittata

Servings: 3
Cooking Time: 45 Minutes
Ingredients:

- 1 stalk celery, diced
- 1/2 (14.5 ounce) can chicken broth
- 1/2 (14-ounce) package seasoned cornbread stuffing mix
- 1/2 cup chopped onion
- 1/4 cup butter
- 1/4 cup water
- 1/4 teaspoon paprika, for garnish
- 2 cups diced cooked ham
- 3 eggs
- 3/4 cup shredded Cheddar cheese

Directions:

1. Lightly grease baking pan of air fryer with cooking spray. Add celery and onions.
2. For 5 minutes, cook on 360°F. Open and stir in ham. Cook for another 5 minutes.
3. Open and stir in butter, water, and chicken broth. Mix well and continue cooking for another 5 minutes.
4. Toss in stuffing mix and toss well to coat. Cover pan with foil.
5. Cook for another 15 minutes.
6. Remove foil and make 3 indentation in the stuffing to hold an egg. Break an egg in each hole.
7. Cook uncovered for another 10 minutes or until egg is cooked to desired doneness.
8. Sprinkle with cheese and paprika. Let it stand in air fryer for another 5 minutes.
9. Serve and enjoy.

161. Mighty Meatballs

Servings: 4
Cooking Time: 20 Minutes
Ingredients:

- 1 egg
- ½ lb. beef minced
- ½ cup friendly breadcrumbs

- 1 tbsp. parsley, chopped
- 2 tbsp. raisins
- 1 cup onion, chopped and fried
- ½ tbsp. pepper
- ½ tsp. salt

Directions:
1. Place all of the ingredients in a bowl and combine well.
2. Use your hands to shape equal amounts of the mixture into small balls. Place each one in the Air Fryer basket.
3. Air fry the meatballs at 350°F for 15 minutes. Serve with the sauce of your choice.

162.Lime Meatballs

Servings: 4
Cooking Time: 7 Minutes
Ingredients:
- ½ teaspoon lime zest, grated
- 1 tablespoon lime juice
- 10 oz ground lamb
- 1 teaspoon ground black pepper
- 1 garlic clove, minced
- ½ teaspoon minced ginger
- 1 teaspoon avocado oil

Directions:
1. In the mixing bowl mix up lime zest, lime juice, ground lamb, minced garlic, and ginger. With the help of the scooper make the meatballs and put them in the freezer for 5-10 minutes. Meanwhile, preheat the air fryer to 380F. Brush the air fryer basket with avocado oil from inside and put the meatballs. Cook them for 7 minutes.

163.Char-grilled Skirt Steak With Fresh Herbs

Servings:3
Cooking Time: 30 Minutes
Ingredients:
- 1 ½ pounds skirt steak, trimmed
- 1 tablespoon lemon zest
- 1 tablespoon olive oil
- 2 cups fresh herbs like tarragon, sage, and mint, chopped
- 4 cloves of garlic, minced
- Salt and pepper to taste

Directions:
1. Preheat the air fryer to 390 °F.
2. Place the grill pan accessory in the air fryer.
3. Season the steak with salt, pepper, lemon zest, herbs, and garlic.
4. Brush with oil.
5. Grill for 15 minutes and if needed cook in batches.

164.New York Steak With Yogurt-cucumber Sauce

Servings:2
Cooking Time: 50 Minutes
Ingredients:
- ½ cup parsley, chopped
- 1 cucumber, seeded and chopped
- 1 cup Greek yogurt
- 2 New York strip steaks
- 3 tablespoons olive oil
- Salt and pepper to taste

Directions:
1. Preheat the air fryer to 390 °F.
2. Place the grill pan accessory in the air fryer.
3. Season the strip steaks with salt and pepper. Drizzle with oil.
4. Grill the steak for 20 minutes per batch and make sure to flip the meat every 10 minutes for even grilling.
5. Meanwhile, combine the cucumber, yogurt, and parsley.

6. Serve the beef with the cucumber yogurt.

165.Leg Of Lamb With Brussels Sprout

Servings:6
Cooking Time:1 Hour 30 Minutes
Ingredients:
- 2¼ pounds leg of lamb
- 1 tablespoon fresh rosemary, minced
- 1 tablespoon fresh lemon thyme
- 1½ pounds Brussels sprouts, trimmed
- 3 tablespoons olive oil, divided
- 1 garlic clove, minced
- Salt and ground black pepper, as required
- 2 tablespoons honey

Directions:
1. Preheat the Air fryer to 300 °F and grease an Air fryer basket.
2. Make slits in the leg of lamb with a sharp knife.
3. Mix 2 tablespoons of oil, herbs, garlic, salt, and black pepper in a bowl.
4. Coat the leg of lamb with oil mixture generously and arrange in the Air fryer basket.
5. Cook for about 75 minutes and set the Air fryer to 390 °F.
6. Coat the Brussels sprout evenly with the remaining oil and honey and arrange them in the Air fryer basket with leg of lamb.
7. Cook for about 15 minutes and dish out to serve warm.

166.Pork Belly Marinated In Onion-coconut Cream

Servings:3
Cooking Time: 25 Minutes
Ingredients:
- ½ pork belly, sliced to thin strips
- 1 onion, diced
- 1 tablespoon butter
- 4 tablespoons coconut cream
- Salt and pepper to taste

Directions:
1. Place all ingredients in a mixing bowl and allow to marinate in the fridge for 2 hours.
2. Preheat the air fryer for 5 minutes.
3. Place the pork strips in the air fryer and bake for 25 minutes at 350 °F.

167.Rosemary Steaks

Servings: 4
Cooking Time: 24 Minutes
Ingredients:
- 4 rib eye steaks
- A pinch of salt and black pepper
- 1 tablespoon olive oil
- 1 teaspoon sweet paprika
- 1 teaspoon cumin, ground
- 1 teaspoon rosemary, chopped

Directions:
1. In a bowl, mix the steaks with the rest of the ingredients, toss and put them in your air fryer's basket. Cook at 380 degrees F for 12 minutes on each side, divide between plates and serve.

168.Sausage And Kale Recipe

Servings: 4
Cooking Time:30 Minutes
Ingredients:
- 1 cup yellow onion; chopped
- 1 ½ lb. Italian pork sausage; sliced
- 1/2 cup red bell pepper; chopped.
- 1/4 cup red hot chili pepper; chopped.
- 1 cup water
- Salt and black pepper to the taste
- 5 lbs. kale; chopped
- 1 tsp. garlic; minced

Directions:

1. In a pan that fits your air fryer, mix sausage with onion, bell pepper, salt, pepper, kale, garlic, water and chili pepper, toss, introduce in preheated air fryer and cook at 300 °F, for 20 minutes. Divide everything on plates and serve.

169.Lamb With Paprika Cilantro Sauce

Servings: 4
Cooking Time: 30 Minutes
Ingredients:

- 1 pound lamb, cubed
- 1 cup coconut cream
- 3 tablespoons sweet paprika
- 2 tablespoons olive oil
- 2 tablespoons cilantro, chopped
- Salt and black pepper to the taste

Directions:

1. Heat up a pan that fits your air fryer with the oil over medium-high heat, add the meat and brown for 5 minutes. Add the rest of the ingredients, toss, put the pan in the air fryer and cook at 380 degrees F for 25 minutes. Divide everything into bowls and serve.

170.Mustard Beef Mix

Servings: 7
Cooking Time: 30 Minutes
Ingredients:

- 2-pound beef ribs, boneless
- 1 tablespoon Dijon mustard
- 1 tablespoon sunflower oil
- 1 teaspoon ground paprika
- 1 teaspoon cayenne pepper

Directions:

1. In the shallow bowl mix up Dijon mustard and sunflower oil. Then sprinkle the beef ribs with ground paprika and cayenne pepper. After this, brush the meat with Dijon mustard mixture and leave for 10 minutes to marinate. Meanwhile, preheat the air fryer to 400F. Put the beef ribs in the air fryer to and cook them for 10 minutes. Then flip the ribs on another side and reduce the air fryer heat to 325F. Cook the ribs for 20 minutes more.

171.Chili Loin Medallions

Servings: 4
Cooking Time: 15 Minutes
Ingredients:

- 1-pound pork loin
- 4 oz bacon, sliced
- 1 teaspoon ground cumin
- 1 teaspoon coconut oil, melted
- ½ teaspoon salt
- ½ teaspoon chili flakes

Directions:

1. Slice the pork loin on the meat medallions and sprinkle them with ground cumin, salt, and chili flakes. Then wrap every meat medallion in the sliced bacon and sprinkle with coconut oil. Place the wrapped medallions in the air fryer basket in one layer and cook them for 10 minutes at 375F. Then carefully flip the meat medallions on another side and cook them for 5 minutes more.

172.Mustard'n Pepper Roast Beef

Servings:9
Cooking Time: 1 Hour And 30 Minutes
Ingredients:

- ¼ cup flat-leaf parsley, chopped
- 1 ½ pounds medium shallots, chopped
- 1 boneless rib roast

- 2 tablespoons whole grain mustard
- 3 tablespoons mixed peppercorns
- 4 medium shallots, chopped
- 4 tablespoons olive oil
- Salt to taste

Directions:
1. Preheat the air fryer for 5 minutes.
2. Place all ingredients in a baking dish that will fit in the air fryer.
3. Place the dish in the air fryer and cook for 1 hour and 30 minutes at 325 °F.

173. Spiced Chops

Servings: 3
Cooking Time: 12 Minutes
Ingredients:
- 10 oz pork chops, bone-in (3 pork chops)
- 1 teaspoon Erythritol
- 1 teaspoon ground black pepper
- 1 teaspoon ground paprika
- ½ teaspoon onion powder
- ¼ teaspoon garlic powder
- 2 teaspoons olive oil

Directions:
1. In the mixing bowl mix up Erythritol, ground black pepper, ground paprika, onion powder, and garlic powder. Then rub the pork chops with the spice mixture from both sides. After this, sprinkle the meat with olive oil. Leave the meat for 5-10 minutes to marinate. Preheat the air fryer to 400F. Put the pork chops in the air fryer and cook them for 6 minutes. Then flip the meat on another side and cook it for 6 minutes more.

174. Cajun 'n Coriander Seasoned Ribs

Servings:4
Cooking Time: 1 Hour

Ingredients:
- ¼ cup brown sugar
- ½ teaspoon lemon
- 1 tablespoon paprika
- 1 tablespoon salt
- 1 teaspoon coriander seed powder
- 2 slabs spareribs
- 2 tablespoons onion powder
- 2 teaspoon Cajun seasoning

Directions:
1. Preheat the air fryer to 390 °F.
2. Place the grill pan accessory in the air fryer.
3. In a small bowl, combine the spaces.
4. Rub the spice mixture on to the spareribs.
5. Place the spareribs on the grill pan and cook for 20 minutes per batch.
6. Serve with your favorite barbecue sauce.

175. Pineapple-teriyaki Beef Skewer

Servings:6
Cooking Time: 12 Minutes
Ingredients:
- 2 tablespoons pineapple juice (optional)
- 2 tablespoons water
- 1 tablespoon vegetable oil
- 1/4 cup and 2 tablespoons light brown sugar
- 1/4 cup soy sauce
- 1-pound boneless round steak, cut into 1/4-inch slices
- 3/4 large garlic cloves, chopped

Directions:
1. In a resealable bag, mix all Ingredients thoroughly except for beef. Then add beef, remove excess air, and seal. Place in ref and marinate for at least a day.

2. Thread beef into skewers and place on skewer rack in air fryer. If needed, cook in batches.
3. For 6 minutes, cook on 390°F.
4. Serve and enjoy.

176.Spicy Lamb Kebabs

Servings:6
Cooking Time:8 Minutes
Ingredients:
- 4 eggs, beaten
- 1 cup pistachios, chopped
- 1 pound ground lamb
- 4 tablespoons plain flour
- 4 tablespoons flat-leaf parsley, chopped
- 2 teaspoons chili flakes
- 4 garlic cloves, minced
- 2 tablespoons fresh lemon juice
- 2 teaspoons cumin seeds
- 1 teaspoon fennel seeds
- 2 teaspoons dried mint
- 2 teaspoons salt
- Olive oil
- 1 teaspoon coriander seeds
- 1 teaspoon freshly ground black pepper

Directions:
1. Preheat the Air fryer to 355 °F and grease an Air fryer basket.
2. Mix lamb, pistachios, eggs, lemon juice, chili flakes, flour, cumin seeds, fennel seeds, coriander seeds, mint, parsley, salt and black pepper in a large bowl.
3. Thread the lamb mixture onto metal skewers to form sausages and coat with olive oil.
4. Place the skewers in the Air fryer basket and cook for about 8 minutes.
5. Dish out in a platter and serve hot.

177.Mustard Lamb Loin Chops

Servings:4
Cooking Time:30 Minutes
Ingredients:
- 8 (4-ounces) lamb loin chops
- 2 tablespoons Dijon mustard
- 1 tablespoon fresh lemon juice
- ½ teaspoon olive oil
- 1 teaspoon dried tarragon
- Salt and black pepper, to taste

Directions:
1. Preheat the Air fryer to 390 °F and grease an Air fryer basket.
2. Mix the mustard, lemon juice, oil, tarragon, salt, and black pepper in a large bowl.
3. Coat the chops generously with the mustard mixture and arrange in the Air fryer basket.
4. Cook for about 15 minutes, flipping once in between and dish out to serve hot.

178.Beef Sausage With Grilled Broccoli

Servings: 4
Cooking Time: 25 Minutes
Ingredients:
- 1 pound beef Vienna sausage
- 1/2 cup mayonnaise
- 1 teaspoon yellow mustard
- 1 tablespoon fresh lemon juice
- 1 teaspoon garlic powder
- 1/4 teaspoon black pepper
- 1 pound broccoli

Directions:
1. Start by preheating your Air Fryer to 380 degrees F. Spritz the grill pan with cooking oil.
2. Cut the sausages into serving sized pieces. Cook the sausages for 15 minutes, shaking the basket

occasionally to get all sides browned. Set aside.

3. In the meantime, whisk the mayonnaise with mustard, lemon juice, garlic powder, and black pepper. Toss the broccoli with the mayo mixture.
4. Turn up temperature to 400 degrees F. Cook broccoli for 6 minutes, turning halfway through the cooking time.
5. Serve the sausage with the grilled broccoli on the side. Bon appétit!

179. Cheesy Schnitzel

Servings: 1
Cooking Time: 30 Minutes
Ingredients:
- 1 thin beef schnitzel
- 1 egg, beaten
- ½ cup friendly bread crumbs
- 2 tbsp. olive oil
- 3 tbsp. pasta sauce
- ¼ cup parmesan cheese, grated
- Pepper and salt to taste

Directions:
1. Pre-heat the Air Fryer to 350°F.
2. In a shallow dish, combine the bread crumbs, olive oil, pepper, and salt. In another shallow dish, put the beaten egg.
3. Cover the schnitzel in the egg before press it into the breadcrumb mixture and placing it in the Air Fryer basket. Cook for 15 minutes.
4. Pour the pasta sauce over the schnitzel and top with the grated cheese. Cook for an additional 5 minutes until the cheese melts. Serve hot.

180. Japanese Miso Steak

Servings: 4

Cooking Time: 15 Minutes + Marinating Time
Ingredients:
- 1 ¼ pounds flank steak
- 1 ½ tablespoons sake
- 1 tablespoon brown miso paste
- 2 garlic cloves, pressed
- 1 tablespoon olive oil

Directions:
1. Place all the ingredients in a sealable food bag; shake until completely coated and place in your refrigerator for at least 1 hour.
2. Then, spritz the steak with a non-stick cooking spray; make sure to coat on all sides. Place the steak in the Air Fryer baking pan.
3. Set your Air Fryer to cook at 400 degrees F. Roast for 12 minutes, flipping twice. Serve immediately.

181. Steak With Bell Peppers

Servings: 4
Cooking Time: 22 Minutes
Ingredients:
- 1¼ pounds beef steak, cut into thin strips
- 2 green bell peppers, seeded and cubed
- 1 red bell pepper, seeded and cubed
- 1 red onion, sliced
- 1 teaspoon dried oregano, crushed
- 1 teaspoon onion powder
- 1 teaspoon garlic powder
- 1 teaspoon red chili powder
- 1 teaspoon paprika
- Salt, to taste
- 2 tablespoons olive oil

Directions:
1. Preheat the Air fryer to 390 °F and grease an Air fryer basket.
2. Mix the oregano and spices in a bowl.

3. Add bell peppers, onion, oil, and beef strips and mix until well combined.
4. Transfer half of the steak strips in the Air fryer basket and cook for about 11 minutes, flipping once in between.
5. Repeat with the remaining mixture and dish out to serve hot.

182.Creamy Pork Chops

Servings: 4
Cooking Time: 10 Minutes
Ingredients:
- 2 pork chops
- ¼ cup coconut flakes
- 3 tablespoons almond flour
- ½ teaspoon salt
- ½ teaspoon dried parsley
- 1 egg, beaten
- 1 tablespoon heavy cream
- 1 teaspoon butter, melted

Directions:
1. Cut every pork chops into 2 chops. Then sprinkle them with salt and dried parsley. After this, in the mixing bowl mix up coconut flakes and almond flour. In the separated bowl mix up egg, heavy cream, and melted butter. Coat the pork chops in the almond flour mixture and them dip in the egg mixture. Repeat the same steps one more time. Then coat the pork chops in the remaining almond flour mixture. Place the meat in the air fryer basket. Cook the pork chops for 10 minutes at 400F. Flip them on another side after 5 minutes of cooking.

183.Simple Lamb Bbq With Herbed Salt

Servings:8
Cooking Time: 1 Hour 20 Minutes
Ingredients:

- 2 ½ tablespoons herb salt
- 2 tablespoons olive oil
- 4 pounds boneless leg of lamb, cut into 2-inch chunks

Directions:
1. Preheat the air fryer to 390 °F.
2. Place the grill pan accessory in the air fryer.
3. Season the meat with the herb salt and brush with olive oil.
4. Grill the meat for 20 minutes per batch.
5. Make sure to flip the meat every 10 minutes for even cooking.

184.Salt And Pepper Pork Chinese Style

Servings:4
Cooking Time: 25 Minutes
Ingredients:
- ½ teaspoon sea salt
- ¾ cup potato starch
- 1 egg white, beaten
- 1 red bell pepper, chopped
- 1 teaspoon Chinese five-spice powder
- 1 teaspoon sesame oil
- 2 green bell peppers, chopped
- 2 tablespoons toasted sesame seeds
- 4 pork chops

Directions:
1. Preheat the air fryer to 330 °F.
2. Season the pork chops with salt and five spice powder.
3. Dip in egg white and dredge in potato starch.
4. Place in the air fryer basket and cook for 25 minutes.
5. Meanwhile, heat oil in a skillet and stir-fry the bell peppers.
6. Serve the bell peppers on top of pork chops and garnish with sesame seeds.

185. Lamb Loin Chops With Lemon

Servings: 4
Cooking Time: 30 Minutes
Ingredients:
- 2 tablespoons Dijon mustard
- 1 tablespoon fresh lemon juice
- ½ teaspoon olive oil
- 1 teaspoon dried tarragon
- Salt and ground black pepper, as required
- 8 (4-ounces) lamb loin chops

Directions:
1. In a large bowl, mix together the mustard, lemon juice, oil, tarragon, salt, and black pepper.
2. Add chops and generously coat with the mixture.
3. Set the temperature of air fryer to 390 degrees F. Grease an air fryer basket.
4. Arrange chops into the prepared air fryer basket in a single layer in 2 batches.
5. Air fry for about 15 minutes, flipping once halfway through.
6. Remove the chops from air fryer and transfer onto serving plates.
7. Serve hot.

186. Filling Pork Chops

Servings: 2
Cooking Time: 12 Minutes
Ingredients:
- 2 (1-inch thick) pork chops
- ½ tablespoon fresh cilantro, chopped
- ½ tablespoon fresh rosemary, chopped
- ½ tablespoon fresh parsley, chopped
- 2 garlic cloves, minced
- 2 tablespoons olive oil
- ¾ tablespoon Dijon mustard
- 1 tablespoon ground coriander
- 1 teaspoon sugar
- Salt, to taste

Directions:
1. Preheat the Air fryer to 390 °F and grease an Air fryer basket.
2. Mix all the ingredients in a large bowl except the chops.
3. Coat the pork chops with marinade generously and cover to refrigerate for about 3 hours.
4. Keep the pork chops at room temperature for about 30 minutes and transfer into the Air fryer basket.
5. Cook for about 12 minutes, flipping once in between and dish out to serve hot.

FISH & SEAFOOD RECIPES

187. Quick-fix Seafood Breakfast

Servings: 2
Cooking Time: 30 Minutes
Ingredients:
- 1 tablespoon olive oil
- 2 garlic cloves, minced
- 1 small yellow onion, chopped
- 1/4 pound tilapia pieces
- 1/4 pound rockfish pieces
- 1/2 teaspoon dried basil
- Salt and white pepper, to taste
- 4 eggs, lightly beaten
- 1 tablespoon dry sherry
- 4 tablespoons cheese, shredded

Directions:
1. Start by preheating your Air Fryer to 350 degrees F; add the olive oil to a baking pan. Once hot, cook the garlic and onion for 2 minutes or until fragrant.
2. Add the fish, basil, salt, and pepper. In a mixing dish, thoroughly combine the eggs with sherry and cheese. Pour the mixture into the baking pan.
3. Cook at 360 degrees F approximately 20 minutes. Bon appétit!

188. Easy Creamy Shrimp Nachos

Servings: 4
Cooking Time: 15 Minutes
Ingredients:
- 1 pound shrimp, cleaned and deveined
- 1 tablespoon olive oil
- 2 tablespoons fresh lemon juice
- 1 teaspoon paprika
- 1/4 teaspoon cumin powder
- 1/2 teaspoon shallot powder
- 1/2 teaspoon garlic powder
- Coarse sea salt and ground black pepper, to taste
- 1 (9-ounce bag corn tortilla chips
- 1/4 cup pickled jalapeño, minced
- 1 cup Pepper Jack cheese, grated
- 1/2 cup sour cream

Directions:
1. Toss the shrimp with the olive oil, lemon juice, paprika, cumin powder, shallot powder, garlic powder, salt, and black pepper.
2. Cook in the preheated Air Fryer at 390 degrees F for 5 minutes.
3. Place the tortilla chips on the aluminum foil-lined cooking basket. Top with the shrimp mixture, jalapeño and cheese. Cook another 2 minutes or until cheese has melted.
4. Serve garnished with sour cream and enjoy!

189. Tarragon And Spring Onions Salmon

Servings: 4
Cooking Time: 15 Minutes
Ingredients:
- 12 oz salmon fillet
- 2 spring onions, chopped
- 1 tablespoon ghee, melted
- 1 teaspoon peppercorns
- ½ teaspoon salt
- ½ teaspoon ground black pepper
- 1 teaspoon tarragon
- ½ teaspoon dried cilantro

Directions:
1. Cut the salmon fillet on 4 servings. Then make the parchment pockets and place the fish fillets in the parchment pockets. Sprinkle the salmon with salt, ground black pepper, tarragon, and dried cilantro.

After this, top the fish with spring onions, peppercorns, and ghee. Preheat the air fryer to 385F. Arrange the salmon pockets in the air fryer in one layer and cook them for 15 minutes.

190.Delicious Crab Cakes

Servings: 4
Cooking Time: 10 Minutes
Ingredients:

- 8 oz crab meat
- 2 tbsp butter, melted
- 2 tsp Dijon mustard
- 1 tbsp mayonnaise
- 1 egg, lightly beaten
- 1/2 tsp old bay seasoning
- 1 green onion, sliced
- 2 tbsp parsley, chopped
- 1/4 cup almond flour
- 1/4 tsp pepper
- 1/2 tsp salt

Directions:

1. Add all ingredients except butter in a mixing bowl and mix until well combined.
2. Make four equal shapes of patties from mixture and place on parchment lined plate.
3. Place plate in the fridge for 30 minutes.
4. Spray air fryer basket with cooking spray.
5. Brush melted butter on both sides of crab patties.
6. Place crab patties in air fryer basket and cook for 10 minutes at 350 F.
7. Turn patties halfway through.
8. Serve and enjoy.

191.Cod And Cauliflower Patties

Servings: 4
Cooking Time: 12 Minutes
Ingredients:

- ½ cup cauliflower, shredded
- 4 oz cod fillet, chopped
- 1 egg, beaten
- 1 teaspoon chives, chopped
- ¼ teaspoon chili flakes
- 1 teaspoon salt
- ½ teaspoon ground cumin
- 2 tablespoons coconut flour
- 1 spring onion, chopped
- 1 tablespoon sesame oil

Directions:

1. Grind the chopped cod fillet and put it in the mixing bowl. Add shredded cauliflower, egg, chives, chili flakes, salt, ground cumin, and chopped onion. Stir the mixture until homogenous and add coconut flour. Stir it again. After this, make the medium size patties. Preheat the air fryer to 385F. Place the patties in the air fryer basket and sprinkle with sesame oil. Cook the fish patties for 8 minutes. Then flip them on another side and cook for 4 minutes more or until the patties are light brown.

192.Air Fried King Prawns

Servings: 4
Cooking Time: 6 Minutes
Ingredients:

- 12 king prawns
- 1 tbsp vinegar
- 1 tbsp ketchup
- 3 tbsp mayonnaise
- 1/2 tsp pepper
- 1 tsp chili powder
- 1 tsp red chili flakes
- 1/2 tsp sea salt

Directions:

1. Preheat the air fryer to 350 F.

2. Spray air fryer basket with cooking spray.
3. Add prawns, chili flakes, chili powder, pepper, and salt to the bowl and toss well.
4. Transfer shrimp to the air fryer basket and cook for 6 minutes.
5. In a small bowl, mix together mayonnaise, ketchup, and vinegar.
6. Serve with mayo mixture and enjoy.

193.Cheese Tilapia

Servings: 4
Cooking Time: 20 Minutes
Ingredients:
- 1 lb. tilapia fillets
- ¾ cup parmesan cheese, grated
- 1 tbsp. parsley, chopped
- 2 tsp. paprika
- 1 tbsp. olive oil
- Pepper and salt to taste

Directions:
1. Pre-heat the Air Fryer to 400°F.
2. In a shallow dish, combine together the paprika, grated cheese, pepper, salt and parsley.
3. Pour a light drizzle of olive oil over the tilapia fillets. Cover the fillets with the paprika and cheese mixture.
4. Lay the fillets on a sheet of aluminum foil and transfer to the Air Fryer basket. Fry for 10 minutes. Serve hot.

194.Calamari

Servings: 2
Cooking Time: 25 Minutes
Ingredients:
- 1 cup club soda
- ½ lb. calamari tubes [or tentacles], about ¼ inch wide, rinsed and dried
- ½ cup honey
- 1 – 2 tbsp. sriracha
- 1 cup flour
- Sea salt to taste
- Red pepper and black pepper to taste
- Red pepper flakes to taste

Directions:
1. 1 In a bowl, cover the calamari rings with club soda and mix well. Leave to sit for 10 minutes.
2. 2 In another bowl, combine the flour, salt, red and black pepper.
3. 3 In a third bowl mix together the honey, pepper flakes, and Sriracha to create the sauce.
4. 4 Remove any excess liquid from the calamari and coat each one with the flour mixture.
5. 5 Spritz the fryer basket with the cooking spray.
6. 6 Arrange the calamari in the basket, well-spaced out and in a single layer.
7. 7 Cook at 380°F for 11 minutes, shaking the basket at least two times during the cooking time.
8. 8 Take the calamari out of the fryer, coat it with half of the sauce and return to the fryer. Cook for an additional 2 minutes.
9. 9 Plate up the calamari and pour the rest of the sauce over it.

195.Sunday's Salmon

Servings: 3
Cooking Time: 20 Minutes
Ingredients:
- ½ lb. salmon fillet, chopped
- 2 egg whites
- 2 tbsp. chives, chopped
- 2 tbsp. garlic, minced
- ½ cup onion, chopped
- 2/3 cup carrots, grated
- 2/3 cup potato, grated
- ½ cup friendly bread crumbs

- ¼ cup flour
- Pepper and salt

Directions:
1. In a shallow dish, combine the bread crumbs with the pepper and salt.
2. Pour the flour into another dish.
3. In a third dish, add the egg whites.
4. Put all of the other ingredients in a large mixing bowl and stir together to combine.
5. Using your hands, shape equal amounts of the mixture into small balls. Roll each ball in the flour before dredging it in the egg and lastly covering it with bread crumbs. Transfer all the coated croquettes to the Air Fryer basket and air fry at 320°F for 6 minutes.
6. Reduce the heat to 350°F and allow to cook for another 4 minutes.
7. Serve hot.

196.Herbed Tuna With Red Onions

Servings: 4
Cooking Time: 20 Minutes
Ingredients:
- 4 tuna steaks
- 1/2 pound red onions
- 4 teaspoons olive oil
- 1 teaspoon dried rosemary
- 1 teaspoon dried marjoram
- 1 tablespoon cayenne pepper
- 1/2 teaspoon sea salt
- 1/2 teaspoon black pepper, preferably freshly cracked
- 1 lemon, sliced

Directions:
1. Place the tuna steaks in the lightly greased cooking basket. Top with the pearl onions; add the olive oil, rosemary, marjoram, cayenne pepper, salt, and black pepper.

2. Bake in the preheated Air Fryer at 400 degrees F for 9 to 10 minutes. Work in two batches.
3. Serve warm with lemon slices and enjoy!

197.Catfish Bites

Servings: 4
Cooking Time: 10 Minutes
Ingredients:
- ¼ cup coconut flakes
- 3 tablespoons coconut flour
- 1 teaspoon salt
- 3 eggs, beaten
- 10 oz catfish fillet
- Cooking spray

Directions:
1. Cut the catfish fillet on the small pieces (nuggets) and sprinkle with salt. After this, dip the catfish pieces in the egg and coat in the coconut flour. Then dip the fish pieces in the egg again and coat in the coconut flakes. Preheat the air fryer to 385F. Place the catfish nuggets in the air fryer basket and cook them for 6 minutes. Then flip the nuggets on another side and cook them for 4 minutes more.

198.Sesame Tuna Steak

Servings: 2
Cooking Time: 12 Minutes
Ingredients:
- 1 tbsp. coconut oil, melted
- 2 x 6-oz. tuna steaks
- ½ tsp. garlic powder
- 2 tsp. black sesame seeds
- 2 tsp. white sesame seeds

Directions:

1. Apply the coconut oil to the tuna steaks with a brunch, then season with garlic powder.
2. Combine the black and white sesame seeds. Embed them in the tuna steaks, covering the fish all over. Place the tuna into your air fryer.
3. Cook for eight minutes at 400°F, turning the fish halfway through.
4. The tuna steaks are ready when they have reached a temperature of 145°F. Serve straightaway.

199.Herbed Trout Mix

Servings: 4
Cooking Time: 20 Minutes
Ingredients:
- 4 trout fillets, boneless and skinless
- 1 tablespoon lemon juice
- 2 tablespoons olive oil
- A pinch of salt and black pepper
- 1 bunch asparagus, trimmed
- 2 tablespoons ghee, melted
- ¼ cup mixed chives and tarragon

Directions:
1. Mix the asparagus with half of the oil, salt and pepper, put it in your air fryer's basket, cook at 380 degrees F for 6 minutes and divide between plates. In a bowl, mix the trout with salt, pepper, lemon juice, the rest of the oil and the herbes and toss, Put the fillets in your air fryer's basket and cook at 380 degrees F for 7 minutes on each side. Divide the fish next to the asparagus, drizzle the melted ghee all over and serve.

200.Sesame Seeds Coated Haddock

Servings:4
Cooking Time:14 Minutes
Ingredients:
- 4 tablespoons plain flour

- 2 eggs
- ½ cup sesame seeds, toasted
- ½ cup breadcrumbs
- 4 (6-ounces) frozen haddock fillets
- 1/8 teaspoon dried rosemary, crushed
- Salt and ground black pepper, as required
- 3 tablespoons olive oil

Directions:
1. Preheat the Air fryer to 390 °F and grease an Air fryer basket.
2. Place the flour in a shallow bowl and whisk the eggs in a second bowl.
3. Mix sesame seeds, breadcrumbs, rosemary, salt, black pepper and olive oil in a third bowl until a crumbly mixture is formed.
4. Coat each fillet with flour, dip into whisked eggs and finally, dredge into the breadcrumb mixture
5. Arrange haddock fillets into the Air fryer basket in a single layer and cook for about 14 minutes, flipping once in between.
6. Dish out the haddock fillets onto serving plates and serve hot.

201.Cornmeal 'n Old Bay Battered Fish

Servings:6
Cooking Time: 15 Minutes
Ingredients:
- ¼ cup flour
- ½ teaspoon garlic powder
- ¾ cup fine cornmeal
- 1 teaspoon paprika
- 2 teaspoons old bay seasoning
- 6 fish fillets cut in half
- Salt and pepper to taste

Directions:
1. Preheat the air fryer to 330 °F.

2. Place the cornmeal, flour, and seasonings in a Ziploc bag.
3. Add the fish fillets and shake until the fish is covered in flour.
4. Place on the double layer rack and cook for 15 minutes.

202.Lemony Tuna-parsley Patties

Servings:4
Cooking Time: 10 Minutes
Ingredients:
- ½ cup panko bread crumbs
- 1 egg, beaten
- 1 tablespoon lemon juice
- 2 cans of tuna in brine
- 2 tablespoons chopped parsley
- 2 teaspoons Dijon mustard
- 3 tablespoons olive oil
- A drizzle Tabasco sauce

Directions:
1. Drain the liquid from the canned tuna and put in a bowl.
2. Mix the tuna and season with mustard, bread crumbs, lemon juice, and parsley.
3. Add the egg and Tabasco sauce. Mix until well combined.
4. Form patties using your hands and place in the fried to set for at least 2 hours.
5. Preheat the air fryer to 390 °F.
6. Place the grill pan accessory.
7. Brush the patties with olive oil and place on the grill pan.
8. Cook for 10 minutes.
9. Make sure to flip the patties halfway through the cooking time for even browning.

203.Cajun Spiced Lemon-shrimp Kebabs

Servings:2
Cooking Time: 10 Minutes
Ingredients:

- 1 tsp cayenne
- 1 tsp garlic powder
- 1 tsp kosher salt
- 1 tsp onion powder
- 1 tsp oregano
- 1 tsp paprika
- 12 pcs XL shrimp
- 2 lemons, sliced thinly crosswise
- 2 tbsp olive oil

Directions:
1. In a bowl, mix all Ingredients except for sliced lemons. Marinate for 10 minutes.
2. Thread 3 shrimps per steel skewer.
3. Place in skewer rack.
4. Cook for 5 minutes at 390°F.
5. Serve and enjoy with freshly squeezed lemon.

204.Fish Packets

Servings: 2
Cooking Time: 15 Minutes
Ingredients:
- 2 cod fish fillets
- 1/2 tsp dried tarragon
- 1/2 cup bell peppers, sliced
- 1/4 cup celery, cut into julienne
- 1/2 cup carrots, cut into julienne
- 1 tbsp olive oil
- 1 tbsp lemon juice
- 2 pats butter, melted
- Pepper
- Salt

Directions:
1. In a bowl, mix together butter, lemon juice, tarragon, and salt. Add vegetables and toss well. Set aside.
2. Take two parchments paper pieces to fold vegetables and fish.
3. Spray fish with cooking spray and season with pepper and salt.
4. Place a fish fillet on each parchment paper piece and top with vegetables.
5. Fold parchment paper around the fish and vegetables.

6. Place veggie fish packets into the air fryer basket and cook at 350 F for 15 minutes.
7. Serve and enjoy.

205.Orange Glazed Scallops

Servings: 3
Cooking Time: 15 Minutes
Ingredients:
- 1 pound jumbo sea scallops
- 1 tablespoon soy sauce
- 2 tablespoons orange juice
- 1 teaspoon orange zest
- 1/2 teaspoon fresh parsley, minced
- 1 tablespoon olive oil
- Sea salt, to taste
- 1/2 teaspoon ground black pepper

Directions:
1. Start by preheating your Air Fryer to 400 degrees F.
2. Toss all ingredients in mixing bowl.
3. Place the scallops in the lightly greased cooking basket and cook for 7 minutes, shaking the basket halfway through the cooking time. Work in batches.
4. Taste, adjust the seasonings and serve warm. Bon appétit!

206.Sautéed Shrimp

Servings:4
Cooking Time: 10 Minutes
Ingredients:
- 1 tbsp olive oil
- ½ a tbsp old bay seasoning
- ¼ a tbsp cayenne pepper
- ¼ a tbsp smoked paprika
- A pinch of sea salt

Directions:
1. Preheat the air fryer to 380 F, and mix all ingredients in a large bowl. Coat the shrimp with a little bit of oil and spices. Place the shrimp in the air fryer's basket and fry for 6-7 minutes. Serve with rice or salad.

207.Almond Sea Bream

Servings: 3
Cooking Time: 10 Minutes
Ingredients:
- 1-pound sea bream steaks (pieces)
- 1 egg, beaten
- 1 tablespoon coconut flour
- 1 teaspoon garlic powder
- 1 tablespoon almond butter, melted
- ½ teaspoon Erythritol
- ½ teaspoon chili powder
- 1 teaspoon apple cider vinegar

Directions:
1. In the shallow bowl mix up garlic powder, coconut flour, chili powder, and Erythritol. Sprinkle the sea bream steaks with apple cider vinegar and dip in the beaten egg. After this, coat every fish steak in the coconut flour mixture. Preheat the air fryer to 390F. Place the fish steak in the air fryer in one layer and sprinkle with almond butter. Cook them for 5 minutes from each side.

208.Homemade Cod Fillets

Servings: 4
Cooking Time: 15 Minutes
Ingredients:
- 4 cod fillets
- ¼ tsp. fine sea salt
- ¼ tsp. ground black pepper, or more to taste
- 1 tsp. cayenne pepper
- ½ cup non-dairy milk
- ½ cup fresh Italian parsley, coarsely chopped
- 1 tsp. dried basil
- ½ tsp. dried oregano
- 1 Italian pepper, chopped
- 4 garlic cloves, minced

Directions:
1. Lightly grease a baking dish with some vegetable oil.
2. Coat the cod fillets with salt, pepper, and cayenne pepper.

3. Blend the rest of the ingredients in a food processor. Cover the fish fillets in this mixture.
4. Transfer the fillets to the Air Fryer and cook at 380°F for 10 to 12 minutes, ensure the cod is flaky before serving.

209.Delicious Snapper En Papillote

Servings: 2
Cooking Time: 20 Minutes
Ingredients:
- 2 snapper fillets
- 1 shallot, peeled and sliced
- 2 garlic cloves, halved
- 1 bell pepper, sliced
- 1 small-sized serrano pepper, sliced
- 1 tomato, sliced
- 1 tablespoon olive oil
- 1/4 teaspoon freshly ground black pepper
- 1/2 teaspoon paprika
- Sea salt, to taste
- 2 bay leaves

Directions:
1. Place two parchment sheets on a working surface. Place the fish in the center of one side of the parchment paper.
2. Top with the shallot, garlic, peppers, and tomato. Drizzle olive oil over the fish and vegetables. Season with black pepper, paprika, and salt. Add the bay leaves.
3. Fold over the other half of the parchment. Now, fold the paper around the edges tightly and create a half moon shape, sealing the fish inside.
4. Cook in the preheated Air Fryer at 390 degrees F for 15 minutes. Serve warm.

210.Broiled Tilapia

Servings: 4
Cooking Time: 10 Minutes

Ingredients:
- 1 lb. tilapia fillets
- ½ tsp. lemon pepper
- Salt to taste

Directions:
1. Spritz the Air Fryer basket with some cooking spray.
2. Put the tilapia fillets in basket and sprinkle on the lemon pepper and salt.
3. Cook at 400°F for 7 minutes.
4. Serve with a side of vegetables.

211.Japanese Ponzu Marinated Tuna

Servings:4
Cooking Time: 10 Minutes

Ingredients:
- 1 cup Japanese ponzu sauce
- 2 tbsp sesame oil
- 1 tbsp red pepper flakes
- 2 tbsp ginger paste
- ¼ cup scallions, sliced
- Salt and black pepper to taste

Directions:
1. In a bowl, mix the ponzu sauce, sesame oil, red pepper flakes, ginger paste, salt, and black pepper. Add in the tuna and toss to coat. Cover and leave to marinate for 60 minutes in the fridge.
2. Preheat air Fryer to 380 F. Spray air fryer basket with cooking spray. Remove tuna from the fridge and arrange on the air fryer basket. Cook for 6 minutes, turning once. Top with scallions to serve.

212.Tuna Au Gratin With Herbs

Servings: 4
Cooking Time: 20 Minutes

Ingredients:
- 1 tablespoon butter, melted
- 1 medium-sized leek, thinly sliced
- 1 tablespoon chicken stock
- 1 tablespoon dry white wine
- 1 pound tuna

- 1/2 teaspoon red pepper flakes, crushed
- Sea salt and ground black pepper, to taste
- 1/2 teaspoon dried rosemary
- 1/2 teaspoon dried basil
- 1/2 teaspoon dried thyme
- 2 small ripe tomatoes, pureed
- 1 cup Parmesan cheese, grated

Directions:
1. Melt 1/2 tablespoon of butter in a sauté pan over medium-high heat. Now, cook the leek and garlic until tender and aromatic. Add the stock and wine to deglaze the pan.
2. Preheat your Air Fryer to 370 degrees F.
3. Grease a casserole dish with the remaining 1/2 tablespoon of melted butter. Place the fish in the casserole dish. Add the seasonings. Top with the sautéed leek mixture.
4. Add the tomato puree. Cook for 10 minutes in the preheated Air Fryer. Top with grated Parmesan cheese; cook an additional 7 minutes until the crumbs are golden. Bon appétit!

213.Crab Cakes

Servings:4
Cooking Time: 55 Minutes
Ingredients:
- ¼ cup chopped red onion
- 1 tbsp chopped basil
- ¼ cup chopped celery
- ¼ cup chopped red pepper
- 3 tbsp mayonnaise
- zest of half a lemon
- ¼ cup breadcrumbs
- 2 tbsp chopped parsley
- Old bay seasoning, as desired
- Cooking spray

Directions:
1. Preheat the air fryer to 390 F.
2. Place all ingredients in a large bowl, and mix well. Make 4 large crab cakes

from the mixture and place them on a lined sheet. Refrigerate for 30 minutes. Spay air basket with cooking spray and arrange the crab cakes inside it. Cook for 7 minutes on each side, until crispy.

214.Peppercorn Cod

Servings: 4
Cooking Time: 15 Minutes
Ingredients:
- 4 cod fillets, boneless
- A pinch of salt and black pepper
- 1 tablespoon thyme, chopped
- ½ teaspoon black peppercorns
- 2 tablespoons olive oil
- 1 fennel, sliced
- 2 garlic cloves, minced
- 1 red bell pepper, chopped
- 2 teaspoons Italian seasoning

Directions:
1. In a bowl, mix the fennel with bell pepper and the other ingredients except the fish fillets and toss. Put this into a pan that fits the air fryer, add the fish on top, introduce the pan in your air fryer and cook at 380 degrees F for 15 minutes. Divide between plates and serve.

215.Spicy Tuna Casserole

Servings: 4
Cooking Time: 20 Minutes
Ingredients:
- 5 eggs, beaten
- 1/2 chili pepper, deveined and finely minced
- 1 ½ tablespoons sour cream
- 1/3 teaspoon dried oregano
- 1/2 tablespoon sesame oil
- 1/3 cup yellow onions, chopped
- 2 cups canned tuna
- 1/2 bell pepper, deveined and chopped
- 1/3 teaspoon dried basil

- Fine sea salt and ground black pepper, to taste

Directions:
1. Warm sesame oil in a nonstick skillet that is preheated over a moderate flame. Then, sweat the onions and peppers for 4 minutes, or until they are just fragrant.
2. Add chopped canned tuna and stir until heated through.
3. Meanwhile, lightly grease a baking dish with a pan spray. Throw in sautéed tuna/pepper mix. Add the remaining ingredients in the order listed above.
4. Bake for 12 minutes at 325 degrees F. Eat warm garnished with Tabasco sauce if desired.

216.Fish Finger Sandwich

Servings:4
Cooking Time: 20 Minutes
Ingredients:
- 2 tbsp flour
- 10 capers
- 4 bread rolls
- 2 oz breadcrumbs
- 4 tbsp pesto sauce
- 4 lettuce leaves
- Salt and pepper, to taste

Directions:
1. Preheat air fryer to 370 F. Season the fillets with salt and pepper, and coat them with the flour; dip in the breadcrumbs. Arrange the fillets onto a baking mat and cook in the fryer for 10 to 15 minutes. Cut the bread rolls in half. Place a lettuce leaf on top of the bottom halves; put the fillets over. Spread a tbsp of pesto sauce on top of each fillet, and top with the remaining halves.

217.Quick Thai Coconut Fish

Servings: 2
Cooking Time: 20 Minutes + Marinating Time
Ingredients:
- 1 cup coconut milk
- 2 tablespoons lime juice
- 2 tablespoons Shoyu sauce
- Salt and white pepper, to taste
- 1 teaspoon turmeric powder
- 1/2 teaspoon ginger powder
- 1/2 Thai Bird's Eye chili, seeded and finely chopped
- 1 pound tilapia
- 2 tablespoons olive oil

Directions:
1. In a mixing bowl, thoroughly combine the coconut milk with the lime juice, Shoyu sauce, salt, pepper, turmeric, ginger, and chili pepper. Add tilapia and let it marinate for 1 hour.
2. Brush the Air Fryer basket with olive oil. Discard the marinade and place the tilapia fillets in the Air Fryer basket.
3. Cook the tilapia in the preheated Air Fryer at 400 degrees F for 6 minutes; turn them over and cook for 6 minutes more. Work in batches.
4. Serve with some extra lime wedges if desired. Enjoy!

SNACKS & APPETIZERS RECIPES

218.Delightful Fish Nuggets

Servings:4
Cooking Time:10 Minutes
Ingredients:
- 1 cup all-purpose flour
- 2 eggs
- ¾ cup breadcrumbs
- 1 pound cod, cut into 1x2½-inch strips
- Pinch of salt
- 2 tablespoons olive oil

Directions:
1. Preheat the Air fryer to 380 °F and grease an Air fryer basket.
2. Place flour in a shallow dish and whisk the eggs in a second dish.
3. Mix breadcrumbs, salt and oil in a third shallow dish.
4. Coat the fish strips evenly in flour and dip in the egg.
5. Roll into the breadcrumbs evenly and arrange the nuggets in an Air fryer basket.
6. Cook for about 10 minutes and dish out to serve warm.

219.Coconut Salmon Bites

Servings: 12
Cooking Time: 10 Minutes
Ingredients:
- 2 avocados, peeled, pitted and mashed
- 4 ounces smoked salmon, skinless, boneless and chopped
- 2 tablespoons coconut cream
- 1 teaspoon avocado oil
- 1 teaspoon dill, chopped
- A pinch of salt and black pepper

Directions:
1. In a bowl, mix all the ingredients, stir well and shape medium balls out of this mix. Place them in your air fryer's basket and cook at 350 degrees F for 10 minutes. Serve as an appetizer.

220.Tofu

Servings: 4
Cooking Time: 20 Minutes
Ingredients:
- 15 oz. extra firm tofu, drained and cut into cubes
- 1 tsp. chili flakes
- ¾ cup cornstarch
- ¼ cup cornmeal
- Pepper to taste
- Salt to taste

Directions:
1. In a bowl, combine the cornmeal, cornstarch, chili flakes, pepper, and salt.
2. Coat the tofu cubes completely with the mixture.
3. Pre-heat your Air Fryer at 350°F.
4. Spritz the basket with cooking spray.
5. Transfer the coated tofu to the basket and air fry for 8 minutes, shaking the basket at the 4-minute mark.

221.The Best Party Mix Ever

Servings: 10
Cooking Time: 15 Minutes
Ingredients:
- 2 cups mini pretzels
- 1 cup mini crackers
- 1 cup peanuts
- 1 tablespoon Creole seasoning
- 2 tablespoons butter, melted

Directions:

1. Toss all ingredients in the Air Fryer basket.
2. Cook in the preheated Air Fryer at 360 degrees F approximately 9 minutes until lightly toasted. Shake the basket periodically. Enjoy!

222.Chocolate Bacon Bites

Servings: 4
Cooking Time: 10 Minutes
Ingredients:
- 4 bacon slices, halved
- 1 cup dark chocolate, melted
- A pinch of pink salt

Directions:
1. Dip each bacon slice in some chocolate, sprinkle pink salt over them, put them in your air fryer's basket and cook at 350 degrees F for 10 minutes. Serve as a snack.

223.Sweet Potato Bites

Servings: 2
Cooking Time: 30 Minutes
Ingredients:
- 2 sweet potatoes, diced into 1-inch cubes
- 1 tsp. red chili flakes
- 2 tsp. cinnamon
- 2 tbsp. olive oil
- 2 tbsp. honey
- ½ cup fresh parsley, chopped

Directions:
1. Pre-heat the Air Fryer at 350°F.
2. Place all of the ingredients in a bowl and stir well to coat the sweet potato cubes entirely.
3. Put the sweet potato mixture into the Air Fryer basket and cook for 15 minutes.

224.Easy And Delicious Pizza Puffs

Servings: 6

Cooking Time: 15 Minutes
Ingredients:
- 6 ounces crescent roll dough
- 1/2 cup mozzarella cheese, shredded
- 3 ounces pepperoni
- 3 ounces mushrooms, chopped
- 1 teaspoon oregano
- 1 teaspoon garlic powder
- 1/4 cup Marina sauce, for dipping

Directions:
1. Unroll the crescent dough. Roll out the dough using a rolling pin; cut into 6 pieces.
2. Place the cheese, pepperoni, and mushrooms in the center of each pizza puff. Sprinkle with oregano and garlic powder.
3. Fold each corner over the filling using wet hands. Press together to cover the filling entirely and seal the edges.
4. Now, spritz the bottom of the Air Fryer basket with cooking oil. Lay the pizza puffs in a single layer in the cooking basket. Work in batches.
5. Bake at 370 degrees F for 5 to 6 minutes or until golden brown. Serve with the marinara sauce for dipping.

225.Loaded Tater Tot Bites

Servings: 6
Cooking Time: 20 Minutes
Ingredients:
- 24 tater tots, frozen
- 1 cup Swiss cheese, grated
- 6 tablespoons Canadian bacon, cooked and chopped
- 1/4 cup Ranch dressing

Directions:
1. Spritz the silicone muffin cups with non-stick cooking spray. Now, press the tater tots down into each cup.

2. Divide the cheese, bacon, and Ranch dressing between tater tot cups.
3. Cook in the preheated Air Fryer at 395 degrees for 10 minutes. Serve in paper cake cups. Bon appétit!

226.Cauliflower Bombs With Sweet & Sour Sauce

Servings: 4
Cooking Time: 25 Minutes
Ingredients:
- Cauliflower Bombs:
- 1/2 pound cauliflower
- 2 ounces Ricotta cheese
- 1/3 cup Swiss cheese
- 1 egg
- 1 tablespoon Italian seasoning mix
- Sweet & Sour Sauce:
- 1 red bell pepper, jarred
- 1 clove garlic, minced
- 1 teaspoon sherry vinegar
- 1 tablespoon tomato puree
- 2 tablespoons olive oil
- Salt and black pepper, to taste

Directions:
1. Blanch the cauliflower in salted boiling water about 3 to 4 minutes until al dente. Drain well and pulse in a food processor.
2. Add the remaining ingredients for the cauliflower bombs; mix to combine well.
3. Bake in the preheated Air Fryer at 375 degrees F for 16 minutes, shaking halfway through the cooking time.
4. In the meantime, pulse all ingredients for the sauce in your food processor until combined. Season to taste. Serve the cauliflower bombs with the Sweet & Sour Sauce on the side. Bon appétit!

227.The Best Calamari Appetizer

Servings: 6
Cooking Time: 20 Minutes
Ingredients:
- 1 ½ pounds calamari tubes, cleaned, cut into rings
- Sea salt and ground black pepper, to taste
- 2 tablespoons lemon juice
- 1 cup cornmeal
- 1 cup all-purpose flour
- 1 teaspoon paprika
- 1 egg, whisked
- 1/4 cup buttermilk

Directions:
1. Preheat your Air Fryer to 390 degrees F. Rinse the calamari and pat it dry. Season with salt and black pepper. Drizzle lemon juice all over the calamari.
2. Now, combine the cornmeal, flour, and paprika in a bowl; add the whisked egg and buttermilk.
3. Dredge the calamari in the egg/flour mixture.
4. Arrange them in the cooking basket. Spritz with cooking oil and cook for 9 to 12 minutes, shaking the basket occasionally. Work in batches.
5. Serve with toothpicks. Bon appétit!

228.Fried Green Tomatoes

Servings: 2
Cooking Time: 10 Minutes
Ingredients:
- 2 medium green tomatoes
- 1 egg
- ¼ cup blanched finely ground flour
- 1/3 cup parmesan cheese, grated

Directions:
1. Slice the tomatoes about a half-inch thick.

2. Crack the egg into a bowl and beat it with a whisk. In a separate bowl, mix together the flour and parmesan cheese.
3. Dredge the tomato slices in egg, then dip them into the flour-cheese mixture to coat. Place each slice into the fryer basket. They may need to be cooked in multiple batches.
4. Cook at 400°F for seven minutes, turning them halfway through the cooking time, and then serve warm.

229.Almond Coconut Granola

Servings:4
Cooking Time: 12 Minutes
Ingredients:
- 1 teaspoon monk fruit
- 1 teaspoon almond butter
- 1 teaspoon coconut oil
- 2 tablespoons almonds, chopped
- 1 teaspoon pumpkin puree
- ½ teaspoon pumpkin pie spices
- 2 tablespoons coconut flakes
- 2 tablespoons pumpkin seeds, crushed
- 1 teaspoon hemp seeds
- 1 teaspoon flax seeds
- Cooking spray

Directions:
1. In the big bowl mix up almond butter and coconut oil. Microwave the mixture until it is melted. After this, in the separated bowl mix up monk fruit, pumpkin spices, coconut flakes, pumpkin seeds, hemp seeds, and flax seeds. Add the melted coconut oil and pumpkin puree. Then stir the mixture until it is homogenous. Preheat the air fryer to 350F. Then put the pumpkin mixture on the baking paper and make the shape of the square. After this, cut the square on the serving bars and transfer in the preheated air fryer. Cook the pumpkin granola for 12 minutes.

230.Mini Cheeseburger Bites

Servings: 4
Cooking Time: 20 Minutes
Ingredients:
- 1 tablespoon Dijon mustard
- 2 tablespoons minced scallions
- 1 pound ground beef
- 1 ½ teaspoons minced green garlic
- 1/2 teaspoon cumin
- Salt and ground black pepper, to savor
- 12 cherry tomatoes
- 12 cubes cheddar cheese

Directions:
1. In a large-sized mixing dish, place the mustard, ground beef, cumin, scallions, garlic, salt, and pepper; mix with your hands or a spatula so that everything is evenly coated.
2. Form into 12 meatballs and cook them in the preheated Air Fryer for 15 minutes at 375 degrees F. Air-fry until they are cooked in the middle.
3. Thread cherry tomatoes, mini burgers and cheese on cocktail sticks. Bon appétit!

231.Tangy Parmesan Chicken Meatballs

Servings: 4
Cooking Time: 15 Minutes
Ingredients:
- 1/2 cup almond flour
- 2 eggs
- 1 ½ tablespoons melted butter
- 1/3 teaspoon mustard seeds
- 1 pound ground chicken
- 2 garlic cloves, finely minced

- 1 teaspoon dried basil
- 1/2 teaspoon Hungarian paprika
- 1/3 cup Parmesan cheese, preferably freshly grated
- 1/2 lime, zested
- 1 teaspoon fine sea salt
- 1/3 teaspoon ground black pepper, or more to taste

Directions:
1. In a nonstick skillet that is preheated over a moderate flame, place the ground chicken and garlic; cook until the chicken is no longer pink and the garlic is just browned, about 3 minutes.
2. Throw in the remaining ingredients; shape the mixture into balls (e.g. the size of a golf ball).
3. Transfer them to the greased Air Fryer cooking basket.
4. Set your Air Fryer to cook at 385 degrees F; cook for about 8 minutes, or till they're thoroughly heated.

232.Mexican Zucchini And Bacon Cakes Ole

Servings: 4
Cooking Time: 22 Minutes
Ingredients:
- 1/3 cup Swiss cheese, grated
- 1/3 teaspoon fine sea salt
- 1/3 teaspoon baking powder
- 1/3 cup scallions, finely chopped
- 1/2 tablespoon fresh basil, finely chopped
- 1 zucchini, trimmed and grated
- 1/2 teaspoon freshly cracked black pepper
- 1 teaspoon Mexican oregano
- 1 cup bacon, chopped
- 1/4 cup almond meal
- 1/4 cup coconut flour

- 2 small eggs, lightly beaten
- 1 cup Cotija cheese, grated

Directions:
1. Mix all ingredients, except for Cotija cheese, until everything is well combined.
2. Then, gently flatten each ball. Spritz the cakes with a nonstick cooking oil.
3. Bake your cakes for 13 minutes at 305 degrees F; work with batches. Serve warm with tomato ketchup and mayonnaise.

233.Banana Chips

Servings: 3
Cooking Time: 20 Minutes
Ingredients:
- 2 large raw bananas, peel and sliced
- ½ tsp. red chili powder
- 1 tsp. olive oil
- ¼ tsp. turmeric powder
- 1 tsp. salt

Directions:
1. Put some water in a bowl along with the turmeric powder and salt.
2. Place the sliced bananas in the bowl and allow to soak for 10 minutes.
3. Dump the contents into a sieve to strain the banana slices before drying them with a paper towel.
4. Pre-heat the Air Fryer to 350°F.
5. Put the banana slices in a bowl and coat them with the olive oil, chili powder and salt.
6. Transfer the chips to the fryer basket and air fry for 15 minutes.

234.Brussels Sprouts

Servings: 2
Cooking Time: 15 Minutes
Ingredients:
- 2 cups Brussels sprouts, sliced in half

- 1 tbsp. balsamic vinegar
- 1 tbsp. olive oil
- ¼ tsp. salt

Directions:

1. Toss all of the ingredients together in a bowl, coating the Brussels sprouts well.
2. Place the sprouts in the Air Fryer basket and air fry at 400°F for 10 minutes, shaking the basket at the halfway point.

235.Coconut Cookies

Servings:8
Cooking Time: 12 Minutes
Ingredients:

- 2¼ ounces caster sugar
- 3½ ounces butter
- 1 small egg
- 1 teaspoon vanilla extract
- 5 ounces self-rising flour
- 1¼ ounces white chocolate, chopped
- 3 tablespoons desiccated coconut

Directions:

1. In a large bowl, add the sugar, and butter and beat until fluffy and light.
2. Add the egg, and vanilla extract and whisk until well combined.
3. Now, add the flour, and chocolate and mix well.
4. In a shallow bowl, place the coconut.
5. With your hands, make small balls from the mixture and roll evenly into the coconut.
6. Place the balls onto an ungreased baking sheet about 1- inch apart and gently, press each ball.
7. Set the temperature of air fryer to 355 degrees F.
8. Place baking sheet into the air fryer basket.
9. Air fry for about 8 minutes and then, another 4 minutes at 320 degrees F.
10. Remove from air fryer and place the baking sheet onto a wire rack to cool for about 5 minutes.
11. Now, invert the cookies onto wire rack to cool completely before serving.
12. Serve.

236.Coconut Radish Chips

Servings: 4
Cooking Time: 15 Minutes
Ingredients:

- 16 ounces radishes, thinly sliced
- A pinch of salt and black pepper
- 2 tablespoons coconut oil, melted

Directions:

1. In a bowl, mix the radish slices with salt, pepper and the oil, toss well, place them in your air fryer's basket and cook at 400 degrees F for 15 minutes, flipping them halfway. Serve as a snack.

237.Cajun Kale Chips

Servings: 4
Cooking Time: 4 Minutes
Ingredients:

- 3 kale heads, cut into pieces
- 2 tbsp Worcestershire sauce
- 2 tbsp sesame oil
- 1 1/2 tsp Cajun spice mix
- Pepper
- Salt

Directions:

1. Add all ingredients into the large bowl and toss well.
2. Transfer kale into the air fryer basket and cook at 195 F for 4-5 minutes.
3. Serve and enjoy.

238.Classic Deviled Eggs

Servings: 3
Cooking Time: 20 Minutes
Ingredients:

- 5 eggs
- 2 tablespoons mayonnaise
- 2 tablespoons sweet pickle relish
- Sea salt, to taste
- 1/2 teaspoon mixed peppercorns, crushed

Directions:

1. Place the wire rack in the Air Fryer basket; lower the eggs onto the wire rack.
2. Cook at 270 degrees F for 15 minutes.
3. Transfer them to an ice-cold water bath to stop the cooking. Peel the eggs under cold running water; slice them into halves.
4. Mash the egg yolks with the mayo, sweet pickle relish, and salt; spoon yolk mixture into egg whites. Arrange on a nice serving platter and garnish with the mixed peppercorns. Bon appétit!

239.Broccoli

Servings: 4
Cooking Time: 30 Minutes
Ingredients:

- 1 large head broccoli
- ½ lemon, juiced
- 3 cloves garlic, minced
- 1 tbsp. coconut oil
- 1 tbsp. white sesame seeds
- 2 tsp. Maggi sauce or other seasonings to taste

Directions:

1. 1 Wash and dry the broccoli. Chop it up into small florets.
2. 2 Place the minced garlic in your Air Fryer basket, along with the coconut oil, lemon juice and Maggi sauce.
3. 3 Heat for 2 minutes at 320°F and give it a stir. Put the garlic and broccoli in the basket and cook for another 13 minutes.
4. 4 Top the broccoli with the white sesame seeds and resume cooking for 5 more minutes, ensuring the seeds become nice and toasty.

240.Yakitori

Servings: 4
Cooking Time: 2 Hours 15 Minutes
Ingredients:

- 1/2 pound chicken tenders, cut bite-sized pieces
- 1 clove garlic, minced
- 1 teaspoon coriander seeds
- Sea salt and ground pepper, to taste
- 2 tablespoons Shoyu sauce
- 2 tablespoons sake
- 1 tablespoon fresh lemon juice
- 1 teaspoon sesame oil

Directions:

1. Place the chicken tenders, garlic, coriander, salt, black pepper, Shoyu sauce, sake, and lemon juice in a ceramic dish; cover and let it marinate for 2 hours.
2. Then, discard the marinade and tread the chicken tenders onto bamboo skewers.
3. Place the skewered chicken in the lightly greased Air Fryer basket. Drizzle sesame oil all over the skewered chicken.
4. Cook at 360 degrees for 6 minutes. Turn the skewered chicken over; brush with the reserved marinade

and cook for a further 6 minutes. Enjoy!

241.Cucumber And Spring Onions Salsa

Servings: 4
Cooking Time: 5 Minutes
Ingredients:

- 1 and ½ pounds cucumbers, sliced
- 2 spring onions, chopped
- 2 tomatoes cubed
- 2 red chili peppers, chopped
- 2 tablespoons ginger, grated
- 1 tablespoon balsamic vinegar
- A drizzle of olive oil

Directions:

1. In a pan that fits your air fryer, mix all the ingredients, toss, introduce in the fryer and cook at 340 degrees F for 5 minutes. Divide into bowls and serve cold as an appetizer.

242.Chinese-style Glazed Baby Carrots

Servings: 6
Cooking Time: 20 Minutes
Ingredients:

- 1 pound baby carrots
- 2 tablespoons sesame oil
- 1/2 teaspoon Szechuan pepper
- 1 teaspoon Wuxiang powder (Five-spice powder)
- 3-4 drops liquid Stevia
- 1 large garlic clove, crushed
- 1 (1-inch) piece fresh ginger root, peeled and grated
- 2 tablespoons tamari sauce

Directions:

1. Start by preheating your Air Fryer to 380 degrees F.
2. Toss all ingredients together and place them in the Air Fryer basket.

3. Cook for 15 minutes, shaking the basket halfway through the cooking time. Enjoy!

243.Vegetable Nuggets

Servings:4
Cooking Time:10 Minutes
Ingredients:

- 1 zucchini, chopped roughly
- ½ of carrot, chopped roughly
- 1 cup all-purpose flour
- 1 egg
- 1 cup panko breadcrumbs
- 1 tablespoon garlic powder
- ½ tablespoon mustard powder
- 1 tablespoon onion powder
- Salt and black pepper, to taste

Directions:

1. Preheat the Air fryer to 380 °F and grease an Air fryer basket.
2. Put zucchini, carrot, mustard powder, garlic powder, onion powder, salt and black pepper in a food processor and pulse until combined.
3. Place flour in a shallow dish and whisk the eggs with milk in a second dish.
4. Place breadcrumbs in a third shallow dish.
5. Coat the vegetable nuggets evenly in flour and dip in the egg mixture.
6. Roll into the breadcrumbs evenly and arrange the nuggets in an Air fryer basket.
7. Cook for about 10 minutes and dish out to serve warm.

244.Crunchy Asparagus With Mediterranean Aioli

Servings: 4
Cooking Time: 50 Minutes
Ingredients:

- Crunchy Asparagus:
- 2 eggs
- 3/4 cup breadcrumbs
- 2 tablespoons Parmesan cheese
- Sea salt and ground white pepper, to taste
- 1/2 pound asparagus, cleaned and trimmed
- Cooking spray
- Mediterranean Aioli:
- 4 garlic cloves, minced
- 4 tablespoons olive oil mayonnaise
- 1 tablespoons lemon juice, freshly squeezed

Directions:
1. Start by preheating your Air Fryer to 400 degrees F.
2. In a shallow bowl, thoroughly combine the eggs, breadcrumbs, Parmesan cheese, salt, and white pepper.
3. Dip the asparagus spears in the egg mixture; roll to coat well. Cook in the preheated Air Fryer for 5 to 6 minutes; work in two batches.
4. Place the garlic on a piece of aluminum foil and spritz with cooking spray. Wrap the garlic in the foil.
5. Cook in the preheated Air Fryer at 400 degrees for 12 minutes. Check the garlic, open the top of the foil and continue to cook for 10 minutes more.
6. Let it cool for 10 to 15 minutes; remove the cloves by squeezing them out of the skins; mash the garlic and add the mayo and fresh lemon juice; whisk until everything is well combined.
7. Serve the asparagus with the chilled aioli on the side. Bon appétit!

245.Zucchini Chips With Greek Dipping Sauce

Servings: 4
Cooking Time: 25 Minutes
Ingredients:
- 1/3 cup almond meal
- 1/2 cup Parmesan cheese, grated
- Sea salt and ground black pepper, to taste
- 1/4 teaspoon oregano
- 1 medium-sized zucchini, cut into slices
- 2 tablespoons grapeseed oil
- Sauce:
- 1/2 cup Greek-style yogurt
- 1 tablespoon fresh cilantro, chopped
- 1 garlic clove, minced
- Freshly ground black pepper, to your liking

Directions:
1. In a shallow bowl, thoroughly combine the almond meal, Parmesan, salt, black pepper, and oregano.
2. Dip the zucchini slices in the prepared batter, pressing to adhere.
3. Brush with the grapeseed oil and cook in the preheated Air Fryer at 400 degrees F for 12 minutes. Shake the Air Fryer basket periodically to ensure even cooking. Work in batches.
4. While the chips are baking, whisk the sauce ingredients; place in your refrigerator until ready to serve. Enjoy!

246.Rangoon Crab Dip

Servings: 8
Cooking Time: 16 Minutes
Ingredients:
- 2 cups crab meat
- 1 cup mozzarella cheese, shredded
- 1/2 tsp garlic powder

- 1/4 cup pimentos, drained and diced
- 1/4 tsp stevia
- 1/2 lemon juice
- 2 tsp coconut amino
- 2 tsp mayonnaise
- 8 oz cream cheese, softened
- 1 tbsp green onion
- 1/4 tsp pepper
- Salt

Directions:

1. Preheat the air fryer to 325 F.
2. Add all ingredients except half mozzarella cheese into the large bowl and mix until well combined.
3. Transfer bowl mixture into the air fryer baking dish and sprinkle with remaining mozzarella cheese.
4. Place into the air fryer and cook for 16 minutes.
5. Serve and enjoy.

247.Coconut Celery Stalks

Servings:4
Cooking Time: 4 Minutes
Ingredients:

- 4 celery stalks
- 1 teaspoon flax meal
- 1 egg, beaten
- 1 teaspoon coconut flour
- 1 teaspoon sunflower oil

Directions:

1. In the bowl mix up flax meal and coconut flour. Then dip the celery stalks in the egg and coat in the flax meal mixture. Sprinkle the celery stalks with sunflower oil and place in the air fryer basket. Cook for 4 minutes at 400F.

248.Lemon Shrimp Bowls

Servings: 4
Cooking Time: 10 Minutes
Ingredients:

- 1 pound shrimp, peeled and deveined
- 3 garlic cloves, minced
- ¼ cup olive oil
- Juice of ½ lemon
- A pinch of salt and black pepper
- ¼ teaspoon cayenne pepper

Directions:

1. In a pan that fits your air fryer, mix all the ingredients, toss, introduce in the fryer and cook at 370 degrees F for 10 minutes. Serve as a snack.

DESSERTS RECIPES

249.Air Fryer Chocolate Cake

Servings:6
Cooking Time:25 Minutes
Ingredients:

- 3 eggs
- 1 cup almond flour
- 1 stick butter, room temperature
- 1/3 cup cocoa powder
- 1½ teaspoons baking powder
- ½ cup sour cream
- 2/3 cup swerve
- 2 teaspoons vanilla

Directions:

1. Preheat the Air fryer to 360 °F and grease a cake pan lightly.
2. Mix all the ingredients in a bowl and beat well.
3. Pour the batter in the cake pan and transfer into the Air fryer basket.
4. Cook for about 25 minutes and cut into slices to serve.

250.Oatmeal Apple & Plum Crumble

Servings: 6
Cooking Time: 20 Minutes
Ingredients:

- ¼ lb. plums, pitted and chopped
- ¼ lb. Braeburn apples, cored and chopped
- 1 tbsp. fresh lemon juice
- 2 ½ oz. sugar
- 1 tbsp. honey
- ½ tsp. ground mace
- ½ tsp. vanilla paste
- 1 cup fresh cranberries
- ⅓ cup oats
- 2/3 cup flour
- ½ stick butter, chilled
- 1 tbsp. cold water

Directions:

1. Coat the plums and apples with the lemon juice, sugar, honey, and ground mace.
2. Lightly coat the inside of a cake pan with cooking spray.
3. Pour the fruit mixture into the pan.
4. In a bowl, mix together all of the other ingredients, combining everything well.
5. Use a palette knife to spread this mixture evenly over the fruit.
6. Place the pan in the Air Fryer and air bake at 390°F for 20 minutes. Ensure the crumble is cooked through before serving.

251.Butter Cake

Servings: 2
Cooking Time: 25 Minutes
Ingredients:

- 1 egg
- 1 ½ cup flour
- 7 tbsp. butter, at room temperature
- 6 tbsp. milk
- 6 tbsp. sugar
- Pinch of sea salt
- Cooking spray
- Dusting of sugar to serve

Directions:

1. Pre-heat the Air Fryer to 360°F.
2. Spritz the inside of a small ring cake tin with cooking spray.
3. In a bowl, combine the butter and sugar using a whisk.
4. Stir in the egg and continue to mix everything until the mixture is smooth and fluffy.
5. Pour the flour through a sieve into the bowl.

6. Pour in the milk, before adding a pinch of salt, and combine once again to incorporate everything well.
7. Pour the batter into the tin and use the back of a spoon to made sure the surface is even.
8. Place in the fryer and cook for 15 minutes.
9. Before removing it from the fryer, ensure the cake is cooked through by inserting a toothpick into the center and checking that it comes out clean.
10. Allow the cake to cool and serve.

252.Classic Buttermilk Biscuits

Servings:4
Cooking Time:8 Minutes
Ingredients:
- ½ cup cake flour
- 1¼ cups all-purpose flour
- ¾ teaspoon baking powder
- ¼ cup + 2 tablespoons butter, cut into cubes
- ¾ cup buttermilk
- 1 teaspoon granulated sugar
- Salt, to taste

Directions:
1. Preheat the Air fryer to 400 °F and grease a pie pan lightly.
2. Sift together flours, baking soda, baking powder, sugar and salt in a large bowl.
3. Add cold butter and mix until a coarse crumb is formed.
4. Stir in the buttermilk slowly and mix until a dough is formed.
5. Press the dough into ½ inch thickness onto a floured surface and cut out circles with a 1¾-inch round cookie cutter.
6. Arrange the biscuits in a pie pan in a single layer and brush butter on them.

7. Transfer into the Air fryer and cook for about 8 minutes until golden brown.

253.Merengues

Servings: 6
Cooking Time: 65 Minutes
Ingredients:
- 2 egg whites
- 1 teaspoon lime zest, grated
- 1 teaspoon lime juice
- 4 tablespoons Erythritol

Directions:
1. Whisk the egg whites until soft peaks. Then add Erythritol and lime juice and whisk the egg whites until you get strong peaks. After this, add lime zest and carefully stir the egg white mixture. Preheat the air fryer to 275F. Line the air fryer basket with baking paper. With the help of the spoon make the small merengues and put them in the air fryer in one layer. Cook the dessert for 65 minutes.

254.Crispy Fruit Tacos

Servings:2
Cooking Time:5 Minutes
Ingredients:
- 2 soft shell tortillas
- 4 tablespoons strawberry jelly
- ¼ cup blueberries
- ¼ cup raspberries
- 2 tablespoons powdered sugar

Directions:
1. Preheat the Air fryer to 300 °F and grease an Air fryer basket.
2. Put 2 tablespoons of strawberry jelly over each tortilla and top with blueberries and raspberries.
3. Sprinkle with powdered sugar and transfer into the Air fryer basket.

4. Cook for about 5 minutes until crispy and serve.

255.All-star Banana Fritters

Servings:5
Cooking Time: 15 Minutes
Ingredients:
- 5 bananas, sliced
- 1 tsp salt
- 3 tbsp sesame seeds
- 1 cup water
- 2 eggs, beaten
- 1 tsp baking powder
- ½ tbsp sugar

Directions:
1. Preheat the air fryer to 340 F.
2. In a bowl, mix salt, sesame seeds, flour, baking powder, eggs, sugar, and water.
3. Coat sliced bananas with the flour mixture; place the prepared slices in the air fryer basket; cook for 8 minutes.

256.Fruity Crumble

Servings:4
Cooking Time:20 Minutes
Ingredients:
- ½ pound fresh apricots, pitted and cubed
- 1 cup fresh blackberries
- 7/8 cup flour
- 1 tablespoon cold water
- ¼ cup chilled butter, cubed
- 1/3 cup sugar, divided
- 1 tablespoon fresh lemon juice
- Pinch of salt

Directions:
1. Preheat the Air fryer to 390 °F and grease a baking pan lightly.

2. Mix apricots, blackberries, 2 tablespoons of sugar and lemon juice in a bowl.
3. Combine the remaining ingredients in a bowl and mix until a crumbly mixture is formed.
4. Pour the apricot mixture in the baking pan and top with the crumbly mixture.
5. Transfer the baking pan in the Air fryer basket and cook for about 20 minutes.
6. Dish out in a bowl and serve warm.

257.Apple Cake

Servings:6
Cooking Time:45 Minutes
Ingredients:
- 1 cup all-purpose flour
- ½ teaspoon baking soda
- 1 egg
- 2 cups apples, peeled, cored and chopped
- 1/3 cup brown sugar
- 1 teaspoon ground nutmeg
- 1 teaspoon ground cinnamon
- Salt, to taste
- 5 tablespoons plus 1 teaspoon vegetable oil
- ¾ teaspoon vanilla extract

Directions:
1. Preheat the Air fryer to 355 °F and grease a baking pan lightly.
2. Mix flour, sugar, spices, baking soda and salt in a bowl until well combined.
3. Whisk egg with oil and vanilla extract in another bowl.
4. Stir in the flour mixture slowly and fold in the apples.
5. Pour this mixture into the baking pan and cover with the foil paper.

6. Transfer the baking pan into the Air fryer and cook for about 40 minutes.
7. Remove the foil and cook for 5 more minutes.
8. Allow to cool completely and cut into slices to serve.

258.Cheesy Orange Fritters

Servings:8
Cooking Time:15 Minutes
Ingredients:
- 1 ½ tablespoons orange juice
- 3/4 pound cream cheese, at room temperature
- 1 teaspoon freshly grated orange rind
- 3/4 cup whole milk
- 1 teaspoon vanilla extract
- 1 ¼ cups all-purpose flour
- 1/3 cup white sugar
- 1/3 teaspoon ground cinnamon
- 1/2 teaspoon ground anise star

Directions:
1. Thoroughly combine all ingredients in a mixing dish.
2. Next step, drop a teaspoonful of the mixture into the air fryer cooking basket; air-fry for 4 minutes at 340 degrees F.
3. Dust with icing sugar, if desired. Bon appétit!

259.Apple Crumble

Servings:4
Cooking Time: 25 Minutes
Ingredients:
- 1 (14-ounces) can apple pie filling
- ¼ cup butter, softened
- 9 tablespoons self-rising flour
- 7 tablespoons caster sugar
- Pinch of salt

Directions:

1. Set the temperature of air fryer to 320 degrees F. Lightly, grease a baking dish.
2. Place apple pie filling evenly into the prepared baking dish.
3. In a medium bowl, add the remaining ingredients and mix until a crumbly mixture forms.
4. Spread the mixture evenly over apple pie filling.
5. Arrange the baking dish in an air fryer basket.
6. Air fry for about 25 minutes.
7. Remove the baking dish from air fryer and place onto a wire rack to cool for about 10 minutes.
8. Serve warm.

260.Baked Coconut Doughnuts

Servings: 6
Cooking Time: 20 Minutes
Ingredients:
- 1 ½ cups all-purpose flour
- 1 teaspoon baking powder
- A pinch of kosher salt
- A pinch of freshly grated nutmeg
- 1/2 cup white sugar
- 2 eggs
- 2 tablespoons full-fat coconut milk
- 2 tablespoons coconut oil, melted
- 1/4 teaspoon ground cardamom
- 1/4 teaspoon ground cinnamon
- 1 teaspoon coconut essence
- 1/2 teaspoon vanilla essence
- 1 cup coconut flakes

Directions:
1. In a mixing bowl, thoroughly combine the all-purpose flour with the baking powder, salt, nutmeg, and sugar.
2. In a separate bowl, beat the eggs until frothy using a hand mixer; add the coconut milk and oil and beat again;

lastly, stir in the spices and mix again until everything is well combined.

3. Then, stir the egg mixture into the flour mixture and continue mixing until a dough ball forms. Try not to over-mix your dough. Transfer to a lightly floured surface.

4. Roll out your dough to a 1/4-inch thickness using a rolling pin. Cut out the doughnuts using a 3-inch round cutter; now, use a 1-inch round cutter to remove the center.

261.Sweet Balls

Servings: 4
Cooking Time: 5 Minutes
Ingredients:
- 1 tablespoon cream cheese
- 3 oz goat cheese
- 2 tablespoons almond flour
- 1 tablespoon coconut flour
- 1 egg, beaten
- 1 tablespoon Splenda
- Cooking spray

Directions:
1. Mash the goat cheese and mix it up with cream cheese. Then add egg, Splenda, and almond flour. Stir the mixture until homogenous. Then make 4 balls and coat them in the coconut flour. Freeze the cheese balls for 2 hours. Preheat the air fryer to 390F. Then place the frozen balls in the air fryer, spray them with cooking spray and cook for 5 minutes or until the cheese balls are light brown.

262.Quick 'n Easy Pumpkin Pie

Servings:8
Cooking Time: 35 Minutes
Ingredients:
- 1 (14 ounce) can sweetened condensed milk

- 1 (15 ounce) can pumpkin puree
- 1 9-inch unbaked pie crust
- 1 large egg
- 1 teaspoon ground cinnamon
- 1/2 teaspoon fine salt
- 1/2 teaspoon ground ginger
- 1/4 teaspoon freshly grated nutmeg
- 1/8 teaspoon Chinese 5-spice powder
- 3 egg yolks

Directions:
1. Lightly grease baking pan of air fryer with cooking spray. Press pie crust on bottom of pan, stretching all the way up to the sides of the pan. Pierce all over with fork.

2. In blender, blend well egg, egg yolks, and pumpkin puree. Add Chinese 5-spice powder, nutmeg, salt, ginger, cinnamon, and condensed milk. Pour on top of pie crust.

3. Cover pan with foil.

4. For 15 minutes, cook on preheated 390°F air fryer.

5. Remove foil and continue cooking for 20 minutes at 330°F until middle is set.

6. Allow to cool in air fryer completely.

7. Serve and enjoy.

263.Favorite Cupcakes With Peanuts

Servings: 8
Cooking Time: 15 Minutes
Ingredients:
- 4 egg whites
- 2 whole egg
- 1/2 teaspoon pure vanilla extract
- 1/2 cup swerve
- 1/2 cup confectioners' swerve
- 1/3 teaspoon cream of tartar
- 1/2 stick butter, softened
- 1/3 teaspoon almond extract
- 1 cup almond flour

- 1/2 cup coconut flour
- 2 tablespoons unsalted peanuts, ground

Directions:
1. First of all, beat the softened butter and swerve until it is fluffy.
2. After that, fold in the egg and mix again; carefully throw in the flour along with ground peanuts; stir in the almond extract and vanilla extract.
3. Divide the batter among the muffin cups that are lined with muffin papers; air-fry at 325 degrees F for 10 minutes.
4. Meanwhile, prepare the topping; simply whip the egg and cream of tartar until it has an airy texture.
5. Now, gradually add the confectioners' swerve; continue mixing until stiff glossy peaks form. To finish, decorate the cupcakes and serve them on a nice serving platter.

264.Brownie Bites

Servings: 16
Cooking Time: 12 Minutes
Ingredients:
- ¾ cup almond flour
- ½ tsp vanilla
- 2 eggs
- ½ cup unsweetened cocoa powder
- ¾ cup swerve
- 4 tbsp butter, melted
- Pinch of salt

Directions:
1. Preheat the air fryer to 325 F.
2. In a bowl, whisk together butter, vanilla, eggs, cocoa powder, sweetener, and salt.
3. Add almond flour and stir to combine.
4. Pour batter into the mini silicone molds and place into the air fryer.

5. Cook for 12 minutes or until done.
6. Serve and enjoy.

265.Strawberry Cheese Cake

Servings: 6
Cooking Time: 35 Minutes
Ingredients:
- 1 cup almond flour
- 3 tbsp coconut oil, melted
- ½ tsp vanilla
- 1 egg, lightly beaten
- 1 tbsp fresh lime juice
- ¼ cup erythritol
- 1 cup cream cheese, softened
- 1 lb strawberries, chopped
- 2 tsp baking powder

Directions:
1. Add all ingredients into the large bowl and mix until well combined.
2. Spray air fryer cake pan with cooking spray.
3. Pour batter into the prepared pan and place into the air fryer and cook at 350 F for 35 minutes.
4. Allow to cool completely.
5. Slice and serve.

266.Easy Fruitcake With Cranberries

Servings: 8
Cooking Time: 30 Minutes
Ingredients:
- 1 cup almond flour
- 1/3 teaspoon baking soda
- 1/3 teaspoon baking powder
- 3/4 cup erythritol
- 1/2 teaspoon ground cloves
- 1/3 teaspoon ground cinnamon
- 1/2 teaspoon cardamom
- 1 stick butter
- 1/2 teaspoon vanilla paste
- 2 eggs plus 1 egg yolk, beaten
- 1/2 cup cranberries, fresh or thawed

- 1 tablespoon browned butter
- For Ricotta Frosting:
- 1/2 stick butter
- 1/2 cup firm Ricotta cheese
- 1 cup powdered erythritol
- 1/4 teaspoon salt
- Zest of 1/2 lemon

Directions:
1. Start by preheating your Air Fryer to 355 degrees F.
2. In a mixing bowl, combine the flour with baking soda, baking powder, erythritol, ground cloves, cinnamon, and cardamom.
3. In a separate bowl, whisk 1 stick butter with vanilla paste; mix in the eggs until light and fluffy. Add the flour/sugar mixture to the butter/egg mixture. Fold in the cranberries and browned butter.
4. Scrape the mixture into the greased cake pan. Then, bake in the preheated Air Fryer for about 20 minutes.
5. Meanwhile, in a food processor, whip 1/2 stick of the butter and Ricotta cheese until there are no lumps.
6. Slowly add the powdered erythritol and salt until your mixture has reached a thick consistency. Stir in the lemon zest; mix to combine and chill completely before using.
7. Frost the cake and enjoy!

267.Fudge Brownies

Servings:8
Cooking Time: 20 Minutes
Ingredients:
- 1 cup sugar
- ½ cup butter, melted
- ½ cup flour
- 1/3 cup cocoa powder
- 1 teaspoon baking powder

- 2 eggs
- 1 teaspoon vanilla extract

Directions:
1. Set the temperature of Air fryer to 350 degrees F. Grease a baking pan.
2. In a large bowl, add the sugar, and butter and whisk until light and fluffy.
3. Add the remaining ingredients and mix until well combined.
4. Place mixture evenly into the prepared pan and with the back of spatula, smooth the top surface.
5. Arrange the baking pan into an air fryer basket.
6. Air fry pan for about 20 minutes.
7. Remove the baking pan from air fryer and set aside to cool completely.
8. Cut into 8 equal-sized squares and serve.

268.Mango Honey Cake

Servings:4
Cooking Time: 50 Minutes
Ingredients:
- 8 oz self-rising flour
- 4 oz butter, softened
- 1 mango, cubed
- ½ cup orange juice
- 1 egg
- 2 tbsp milk
- ½ cup honey

Directions:
1. Preheat air fryer to 390 F. In a bowl, mix butter and flour. Crumble the mixture with your fingers. Stir in mango, honey, chocolate, and juice. Whisk egg and milk in another bowl, and then add to the batter. Transfer the batter to a greased cake pan, put in the air fryer, and cook for 40 minutes. Let cool before serving.

269.Simple Donuts

Servings:12
Cooking Time:25 Minutes
Ingredients:
- 2 cups all-purpose flour
- 2 teaspoons baking powder
- 1 egg
- 1 tablespoon butter, softened
- ½ cup milk
- Salt, to taste
- ¾ cup sugar
- 2 teaspoons vanilla extract
- 2 tablespoons icing sugar

Directions:
1. Preheat the Air fryer to 390 °F and grease an Air fryer basket lightly.
2. Sift together flour, baking powder and salt in a large bowl.
3. Add sugar and egg and mix well.
4. Stir in the butter, milk and vanilla extract and mix until a dough is formed.
5. Refrigerate the dough for at least 1 hour and roll the dough into ½ inch thickness onto a floured surface.
6. Cut into donuts with a donut cutter and arrange the donuts in the Air fryer basket in 3 batches.
7. Cook for about 8 minutes until golden and serve.

270.Baked Peaches With Oatmeal Pecan Streusel

Servings: 3
Cooking Time: 20 Minutes
Ingredients:
- 2 tablespoons old-fashioned rolled oats
- 3 tablespoons golden caster sugar
- 1/2 teaspoon ground cinnamon
- 1 egg
- 2 tablespoons cold salted butter, cut into pieces
- 3 tablespoons pecans, chopped
- 3 large ripe freestone peaches, halved and pitted

Directions:
1. Mix the rolled oats, sugar, cinnamon, egg, and butter until well combined.
2. Add a big spoonful of prepared topping to the center of each peach. Pour 1/2 cup of water into an Air Fryer safe dish. Place the peaches in the dish.
3. Top the peaches with the roughly chopped pecans. Bake at 340 degrees F for 17 minutes. Serve at room temperature. Bon appétit!

271.Coconut 'n Almond Fat Bombs

Servings:12
Cooking Time: 15 Minutes
Ingredients:
- ¼ cup almond flour
- ½ cup shredded coconut
- 1 tablespoon coconut oil
- 1 tablespoon vanilla extract
- 2 tablespoons liquid stevia
- 3 egg whites

Directions:
1. Preheat the air fryer for 5 minutes.
2. Combine all ingredients in a mixing bowl.
3. Form small balls using your hands.
4. Place in the air fryer basket and cook for 15 minutes at 400 °F.

272.Pumpkin Muffins

Servings: 10
Cooking Time: 20 Minutes
Ingredients:
- 4 large eggs
- 1/2 cup pumpkin puree

- 1 tbsp pumpkin pie spice
- 1 tbsp baking powder, gluten-free
- 2/3 cup erythritol
- 1 tsp vanilla
- 1/3 cup coconut oil, melted
- 1/2 cup almond flour
- 1/2 cup coconut flour
- 1/2 tsp sea salt

Directions:
1. Preheat the air fryer to 325 F.
2. In a large bowl, stir together coconut flour, pumpkin pie spice, baking powder, erythritol, almond flour, and sea salt.
3. Stir in eggs, vanilla, coconut oil, and pumpkin puree until well combined.
4. Pour batter into the silicone muffin molds and place into the air fryer basket in batches.
5. Cook muffins for 20 minutes.
6. Serve and enjoy.

273.Pecan Muffins

Servings: 12
Cooking Time: 15 Minutes
Ingredients:
- 4 eggs
- 1 tsp vanilla
- 1/4 cup almond milk
- 2 tbsp butter, melted
- 1/2 cup swerve
- 1 tsp psyllium husk
- 1 tbsp baking powder
- 1/2 cup pecans, chopped
- 1/2 tsp ground cinnamon
- 2 tsp allspice
- 1 1/2 cups almond flour

Directions:
1. Preheat the air fryer to 370 F.
2. Beat eggs, almond milk, vanilla, sweetener, and butter in a bowl using a hand mixer until smooth.

3. Add remaining ingredients and mix until well combined.
4. Pour batter into the silicone muffin molds and place into the air fryer basket in batches.
5. Cook muffins for 15 minutes.
6. Serve and enjoy.

274.Chocolate Cookies

Servings: 8
Cooking Time: 30 Minutes
Ingredients:
- 3 oz. sugar
- 4 oz. butter
- 1 tbsp. honey
- 6 oz. flour
- 1 ½ tbsp. milk
- 2 oz. chocolate chips

Directions:
1. Pre-heat the Air Fryer to 350°F.
2. Mix together the sugar and butter using an electric mixer, until a fluffy texture is achieved.
3. Stir in the remaining ingredients, minus the chocolate chips.
4. Gradually fold in the chocolate chips.
5. Spoon equal portions of the mixture onto a lined baking sheet and flatten out each one with a spoon. Ensure the cookies are not touching.
6. Place in the fryer and cook for 18 minutes.

275.Tasty Lemony Biscuits

Servings:10
Cooking Time:5 Minutes
Ingredients:
- 8½ ounce self-rising flour
- 3½-ounce cold butter
- 1 small egg
- 1 teaspoon fresh lemon zest, grated finely

- 3½-ounce caster sugar
- 2 tablespoons fresh lemon juice
- 1 teaspoon vanilla extract

Directions:

1. Preheat the Air fryer to 355 °F and grease a baking sheet lightly.
2. Mix flour and sugar in a large bowl.
3. Add cold butter and mix until a coarse crumb is formed.
4. Stir in the egg, lemon zest and lemon juice and mix until a dough is formed.
5. Press the dough into ½ inch thickness onto a floured surface and cut dough into medium-sized biscuits.
6. Arrange the biscuits on a baking sheet in a single layer and transfer into the Air fryer.
7. Cook for about 5 minutes until golden brown and serve with tea.

276.Zucchinis Bars

Servings: 12
Cooking Time: 15 Minutes

Ingredients:

- 3 tablespoons coconut oil, melted
- 6 eggs
- 3 ounces zucchini, shredded
- 2 teaspoons vanilla extract
- ½ teaspoon baking powder
- 4 ounces cream cheese
- 2 tablespoons erythritol

Directions:

1. In a bowl, combine all the ingredients and whisk well. pour this into a baking dish that fits your air fryer lined with parchment paper, introduce in the fryer and cook at 320 degrees F, bake for 15 minutes. Slice and serve cold.

277.Semolina Cake

Servings:8

Cooking Time:15 Minutes

Ingredients:

- 2½ cups semolina
- 1 cup milk
- 1 cup Greek yogurt
- 2 teaspoons baking powder
- ½ cup walnuts, chopped
- ½ cup vegetable oil
- 1 cup sugar
- Pinch of salt

Directions:

1. Preheat the Air fryer to 360 °F and grease a baking pan lightly.
2. Mix semolina, oil, milk, yogurt and sugar in a bowl until well combined.
3. Cover the bowl and keep aside for about 15 minutes.
4. Stir in the baking soda, baking powder and salt and fold in the walnuts.
5. Transfer the mixture into the baking pan and place in the Air fryer.
6. Cook for about 15 minutes and dish out to serve.

278.Chocolate Coffee Cake

Servings: 8
Cooking Time: 40 Minutes

Ingredients:

- 1 ½ cups almond flour
- 1/2 cup coconut meal
- 2/3 cup swerve
- 1 teaspoon baking powder
- 1/4 teaspoon salt
- 1 stick butter, melted
- 1/2 cup hot strongly brewed coffee
- 1/2 teaspoon vanilla
- 1 egg
- Topping:
- 1/4 cup coconut flour
- 1/2 cup confectioner's swerve
- 1/2 teaspoon ground cardamom

- 1 teaspoon ground cinnamon
- 3 tablespoons coconut oil

Directions:

1. Mix all dry ingredients for your cake; then, mix in the wet ingredients. Mix until everything is well incorporated.
2. Spritz a baking pan with cooking spray. Scrape the batter into the baking pan.
3. Then, make the topping by mixing all ingredients. Place on top of the cake. Smooth the top with a spatula.
4. Bake at 330 degrees F for 30 minutes or until the top of the cake springs back when gently pressed with your fingers. Serve with your favorite hot beverage. Bon appétit!

279. Macaroon Bites

Servings: 2
Cooking Time: 30 Minutes
Ingredients:

- 4 egg whites
- ½ tsp vanilla
- ½ tsp EZ-Sweet (or equivalent of 1 cup artificial sweetener)
- 4½ tsp water
- 1 cup unsweetened coconut

Directions:

1. Preheat your fryer to 375°F/190°C.
2. Combine the egg whites, liquids and coconut.
3. Put into the fryer and reduce the heat to 325°F/160°C.
4. Bake for 15 minutes.
5. Serve!

OTHER AIR FRYER RECIPES

280.Greek Omelet With Halloumi Cheese

Servings: 2
Cooking Time: 17 Minutes
Ingredients:

- 1/2 cup Halloumi cheese, sliced
- 2 teaspoons garlic paste
- 2 teaspoons fresh chopped rosemary
- 4well-whisked eggs
- 2 bell peppers, seeded and chopped
- 1 ½ tablespoons fresh basil, chopped
- 3 tablespoons onions, chopped
- Fine sea salt and ground black pepper, to taste

Directions:

1. Spritz your baking dish with a canola cooking spray.
2. Throw in all ingredients and stir until everything is well incorporated.
3. Bake for about 15 minutes at 325 degrees F. Eat warm.

281.Veggie Casserole With Ham And Baked Eggs

Servings: 4
Cooking Time: 30 Minutes
Ingredients:

- 2 tablespoons butter, melted
- 1 zucchini, diced
- 1 bell pepper, seeded and sliced
- 1 red chili pepper, seeded and minced
- 1 medium-sized leek, sliced
- 3/4 pound ham, cooked and diced
- 5 eggs
- 1 teaspoon cayenne pepper
- Sea salt, to taste
- 1/2 teaspoon ground black pepper
- 1 tablespoon fresh cilantro, chopped

Directions:

1. Start by preheating the Air Fryer to 380 degrees F. Grease the sides and bottom of a baking pan with the melted butter.
2. Place the zucchini, peppers, leeks and ham in the baking pan. Bake in the preheated Air Fryer for 6 minutes.
3. Crack the eggs on top of ham and vegetables; season with the cayenne pepper, salt, and black pepper. Bake for a further 20 minutes or until the whites are completely set.
4. Garnish with fresh cilantro and serve. Bon appétit!

282.Spicy Peppery Egg Salad

Servings: 3
Cooking Time: 20 Minutes + Chilling Time
Ingredients:

- 6 eggs
- 1 teaspoon mustard
- 1/2 cup mayonnaise
- 1 tablespoon white vinegar
- 1 habanero pepper, minced
- 1 red bell pepper, seeded and sliced
- 1 green bell pepper, seeded and sliced
- 1 shallot, sliced
- Sea salt and ground black pepper, to taste

Directions:

1. Place the wire rack in the Air Fryer basket; lower the eggs onto the wire rack.
2. Cook at 270 degrees F for 15 minutes.
3. Transfer them to an ice-cold water bath to stop the cooking. Peel the eggs under cold running water; coarsely chop the hard-boiled eggs and set aside.
4. Toss with the remaining ingredients and serve well chilled. Bon appétit!

283.Jamaican Cornmeal Pudding

Servings: 6
Cooking Time: 1 Hour + Chilling Time
Ingredients:

- 3 cups coconut milk
- 2 ounces butter, softened
- 1 teaspoon cinnamon
- 1/2 teaspoon grated nutmeg
- 1 cup sugar
- 1/2 teaspoon fine sea salt
- 1 ½ cups yellow cornmeal
- 1/4 cup all-purpose flour
- 1/2 cup water
- 1/2 cup raisins
- 1 teaspoon rum extract
- 1 teaspoon vanilla extract
- Custard:
- 1/2 cup full-fat coconut milk
- 1 ounce butter
- 1/4 cup honey
- 1 dash vanilla

Directions:

1. Place the coconut milk, butter, cinnamon, nutmeg, sugar, and salt in a large saucepan; bring to a rapid boil. Heat off.
2. In a mixing bowl, thoroughly combine the cornmeal, flour and water; mix to combine well.
3. Add the milk/butter mixture to the cornmeal mixture; mix to combine. Bring the cornmeal mixture to boil; then, reduce the heat and simmer approximately 7 minutes, whisking continuously.
4. Remove from the heat. Now, add the raisins, rum extract, and vanilla.
5. Place the mixture into a lightly greased baking pan and bake at 325 degrees F for 12 minutes.
6. In a saucepan, whisk the coconut milk, butter, honey, and vanilla; let it simmer for 2 to 3 minutes. Now, prick your pudding with a fork and top with the prepared custard.
7. Return to your Air Fryer and bake for about 35 minutes more or until a toothpick inserted comes out dry and clean. Place in your refrigerator until ready to serve. Bon appétit!

284.Tangy Paprika Chicken

Servings: 4
Cooking Time: 30 Minutes
Ingredients:

- 1 ½ tablespoons freshly squeezed lemon juice
- 2 small-sized chicken breasts, boneless
- 1/2 teaspoon ground cumin
- 1 teaspoon dry mustard powder
- 1 teaspoon paprika
- 2 teaspoons cup pear cider vinegar
- 1 tablespoon olive oil
- 2 garlic cloves, minced
- Kosher salt and freshly ground mixed peppercorns, to savor

Directions:

1. Warm the olive oil in a nonstick pan over a moderate flame. Sauté the garlic for just 1 minutes.
2. Remove your pan from the heat; add cider vinegar, lemon juice, paprika, cumin, mustard powder, kosher salt, and black pepper. Pour this paprika sauce into a baking dish.
3. Pat the chicken breasts dry; transfer them to the prepared sauce. Bake in the preheated air fryer for about 28 minutes at 335 degrees F; check for doneness using a thermometer or a fork.

4. Allow to rest for 8 to 9 minutes before slicing and serving. Serve with dressing.

285.Breakfast Eggs With Swiss Chard And Ham

Servings: 2
Cooking Time: 20 Minutes
Ingredients:
- 2 eggs
- 1/4 teaspoon dried or fresh marjoram
- 2 teaspoons chili powder
- 1/3 teaspoon kosher salt
- 1/2 cup steamed Swiss Chard
- 1/4 teaspoon dried or fresh rosemary
- 4 pork ham slices
- 1/3 teaspoon ground black pepper, or more to taste

Directions:
1. Divide the Swiss Chard and ham among 2 ramekins; crack an egg into each ramekin. Sprinkle with seasonings.
2. Cook for 15 minutes at 335 degrees F or until your eggs reach desired texture.
3. Serve warm with spicy tomato ketchup and pickles. Bon appétit!

286.Baked Eggs Florentine

Servings: 2
Cooking Time: 20 Minutes
Ingredients:
- 1 tablespoon ghee, melted
- 2 cups baby spinach, torn into small pieces
- 2 tablespoons shallots, chopped
- 1/4 teaspoon red pepper flakes
- Salt, to taste
- 1 tablespoon fresh thyme leaves, roughly chopped

- 4 eggs

Directions:
1. Start by preheating your Air Fryer to 350 degrees F. Brush the sides and bottom of a gratin dish with the melted ghee.
2. Put the spinach and shallots into the bottom of the gratin dish. Season with red pepper, salt, and fresh thyme.
3. Make four indents for the eggs; crack one egg into each indent. Bake for 12 minutes, rotating the pan once or twice to ensure even cooking. Enjoy!

287.The Best London Broil Ever

Servings: 8
Cooking Time: 30 Minutes + Marinating Time
Ingredients:
- 2 pounds London broil
- 3 large garlic cloves, minced
- 3 tablespoons balsamic vinegar
- 3 tablespoons whole-grain mustard
- 2 tablespoons olive oil
- Sea salt and ground black pepper, to taste
- 1/2 teaspoon dried hot red pepper flakes

Directions:
1. Score both sides of the cleaned London broil.
2. Thoroughly combine the remaining ingredients; massage this mixture into the meat to coat it on all sides. Let it marinate for at least 3 hours.
3. Set the Air Fryer to cook at 400 degrees F; Then cook the London broil for 15 minutes. Flip it over and cook another 10 to 12 minutes. Bon appétit!

288.Grilled Lemony Pork Chops

Servings: 5
Cooking Time: 34 Minutes

Ingredients:

- 5 pork chops
- 1/3 cup vermouth
- 1/2 teaspoon paprika
- 2 sprigs thyme, only leaves, crushed
- 1/2 teaspoon dried oregano
- Fresh parsley, to serve
- 1 teaspoon garlic salt½ lemon, cut into wedges
- 1 teaspoon freshly cracked black pepper
- 3 tablespoons lemon juice
- 3 cloves garlic, minced
- 2 tablespoons canola oil

Directions:

1. Firstly, heat the canola oil in a sauté pan over a moderate heat. Now, sweat the garlic until just fragrant.
2. Remove the pan from the heat and pour in the lemon juice and vermouth. Now, throw in the seasonings. Dump the sauce into a baking dish, along with the pork chops.
3. Tuck the lemon wedges among the pork chops and air-fry for 27 minutes at 345 degrees F. Bon appétit!

289.Delicious Hot Fruit Bake

Servings: 4
Cooking Time: 40 Minutes
Ingredients:

- 2 cups blueberries
- 2 cups raspberries
- 1 tablespoon cornstarch
- 3 tablespoons maple syrup
- 2 tablespoons coconut oil, melted
- A pinch of freshly grated nutmeg
- A pinch of salt
- 1 cinnamon stick
- 1 vanilla bean

Directions:

1. Place your berries in a lightly greased baking dish. Sprinkle the cornstarch onto the fruit.
2. Whisk the maple syrup, coconut oil, nutmeg, and salt in a mixing dish; add this mixture to the berries and gently stir to combine.
3. Add the cinnamon and vanilla. Bake in the preheated Air Fryer at 370 degrees F for 35 minutes. Serve warm or at room temperature. Enjoy!

290.Gorgonzola Stuffed Mushrooms With Horseradish Mayo

Servings: 5
Cooking Time: 15 Minutes
Ingredients:

- 1/2 cup of breadcrumbs
- 2 cloves garlic, pressed
- 2 tablespoons fresh coriander, chopped
- 1/3 teaspoon kosher salt
- 1/2 teaspoon crushed red pepper flakes
- 1 ½ tablespoons olive oil
- 20 medium-sized mushrooms, cut off the stems
- 1/2 cup Gorgonzola cheese, grated
- 1/4 cup low-fat mayonnaise
- 1 teaspoon prepared horseradish, well-drained
- 1 tablespoon fresh parsley, finely chopped

Directions:

1. Mix the breadcrumbs together with the garlic, coriander, salt, red pepper, and the olive oil; mix to combine well.
2. Stuff the mushroom caps with the breadcrumb filling. Top with grated Gorgonzola.
3. Place the mushrooms in the Air Fryer grill pan and slide them into the

machine. Grill them at 380 degrees F for 8 to 12 minutes or until the stuffing is warmed through.

4. Meanwhile, prepare the horseradish mayo by mixing the mayonnaise, horseradish and parsley. Serve with the warm fried mushrooms. Enjoy!

291.Greek Frittata With Feta Cheese

Servings: 4
Cooking Time: 10 Minutes
Ingredients:
- 1/3 cup Feta cheese, crumbled
- 1 teaspoon dried rosemary
- 2 tablespoons fish sauce
- 1 ½ cup cooked chicken breasts, boneless and shredded
- 1/2 teaspoon coriander sprig, finely chopped
- 6 medium-sized whisked eggs
- 1/3 teaspoon ground white pepper
- 1 cup fresh chives, chopped
- 1/2 teaspoon garlic paste
- Fine sea salt, to taste
- Nonstick cooking spray

Directions:
1. Grab a baking dish that fit in your Air Fryer.
2. Lightly coat the inside of the baking dish with a nonstick cooking spray of choice. Stir in all ingredients, minus feta cheese. Stir to combine well.
3. Set your Air Fryer to cook at 335 degrees for 8 minutes; check for doneness. Scatter crumbled feta over the top and eat immediately!

292.Sweet Mini Monkey Rolls

Servings: 6
Cooking Time: 25 Minutes
Ingredients:
- 3/4 cup brown sugar

- 1 stick butter, melted
- 1/4 cup granulated sugar
- 1 teaspoon ground cinnamon
- 1/4 teaspoon ground cardamom
- 1 (16-ounce) can refrigerated buttermilk biscuit dough

Directions:
1. Spritz 6 standard-size muffin cups with nonstick spray. Mix the brown sugar and butter; divide the mixture between muffin cups.
2. Mix the granulated sugar with cinnamon and cardamom. Separate the dough into 16 biscuits; cut each in 6 pieces. Roll the pieces over the cinnamon sugar mixture to coat. Divide between muffin cups.
3. Bake at 340 degrees F for about 20 minutes or until golden brown. Turn upside down and serve.

293.Cheddar Cheese And Pastrami Casserole

Servings: 2
Cooking Time: 20 Minutes
Ingredients:
- 4 eggs
- 1 bell pepper, chopped
- 2 spring onions, chopped
- 1 cup pastrami, sliced
- 1/4 cup Greek-style yogurt
- 1/2 cup Cheddar cheese, grated
- Sea salt, to taste
- 1/4 teaspoon ground black pepper

Directions:
1. Start by preheating your Air Fryer to 330 degrees F. Spritz the baking pan with cooking oil.
2. Then, thoroughly combine all ingredients and pour the mixture into the prepared baking pan.

3. Cook for 7 to 9 minutes or until the eggs have set. Place on a cooling rack and let it sit for 10 minutes before slicing and serving.

294.Zesty Broccoli Bites With Hot Sauce

Servings: 6
Cooking Time: 20 Minutes
Ingredients:
- For the Broccoli Bites:
- 1 medium-sized head broccoli, broken into florets
- 1/2 teaspoon lemon zest, freshly grated
- 1/3 teaspoon fine sea salt
- 1/2 teaspoon hot paprika
- 1 teaspoon shallot powder
- 1 teaspoon porcini powder
- 1/2 teaspoon granulated garlic
- 1/3 teaspoon celery seeds
- 1 ½ tablespoons olive oil
- For the Hot Sauce:
- 1/2 cup tomato sauce
- 3 tablespoons brown sugar
- 1 tablespoon balsamic vinegar
- 1/2 teaspoon ground allspice

Directions:
1. Toss all the ingredients for the broccoli bites in a mixing bowl, covering the broccoli florets on all sides.
2. Cook them in the preheated Air Fryer at 360 degrees for 13 to 15 minutes. In the meantime, mix all ingredients for the hot sauce.
3. Pause your Air Fryer, mix the broccoli with the prepared sauce and cook for further 3 minutes. Bon appétit!

295.Turkey Wontons With Garlic-parmesan Sauce

Servings: 8

Cooking Time: 15 Minutes
Ingredients:
- 8 ounces cooked turkey breasts, shredded
- 16 wonton wrappers
- 1 ½ tablespoons butter, melted
- 1/3 cup cream cheese, room temperature
- 8 ounces Asiago cheese, shredded
- 3 tablespoons Parmesan cheese, grated
- 1 teaspoon garlic powder
- Fine sea salt and freshly ground black pepper, to taste

Directions:
1. In a small-sized bowl, mix the butter, Parmesan, garlic powder, salt, and black pepper; give it a good stir.
2. Lightly grease a mini muffin pan; lay 1 wonton wrapper in each mini muffin cup. Fill each cup with the cream cheese and turkey mixture.
3. Air-fry for 8 minutes at 335 degrees F. Immediately top with Asiago cheese and serve warm. Bon appétit!

296.Potato Appetizer With Garlic-mayo Sauce

Servings: 4
Cooking Time: 19 Minutes
Ingredients:
- 2 tablespoons vegetable oil of choice
- Kosher salt and freshly ground black pepper, to taste
- 3 Russet potatoes, cut into wedges
- For the Dipping Sauce:
- 2 teaspoons dried rosemary, crushed
- 3 garlic cloves, minced
- 1/3 teaspoon dried marjoram, crushed
- 1/4 cup sour cream
- 1/3 cup mayonnaise

Directions:

1. Lightly grease your potatoes with a thin layer of vegetable oil. Season with salt and ground black pepper.
2. Arrange the seasoned potato wedges in an air fryer cooking basket. Bake at 395 degrees F for 15 minutes, shaking once or twice.
3. In the meantime, prepare the dipping sauce by mixing all the sauce ingredients. Serve the potatoes with the dipping sauce and enjoy!

297. Za'atar Eggs With Chicken And Provolone Cheese

Servings: 2
Cooking Time: 20 Minutes
Ingredients:

- 1/3 cup milk
- 1 1/2 Roma tomato, chopped
- 1/3 cup Provolone cheese, grated
- 1 teaspoon freshly cracked pink peppercorns
- 3 eggs
- 1 teaspoon Za'atar
- ½ chicken breast, cooked
- 1 teaspoon fine sea salt
- 1 teaspoon freshly cracked pink peppercorns

Directions:

1. Preheat your air fryer to cook at 365 degrees F. In a medium-sized mixing dish, whisk the eggs together with the milk, Za'atar, sea salt, and cracked pink peppercorns.
2. Spritz the ramekins with cooking oil; divide the prepared egg mixture among the greased ramekins.
3. Shred the chicken with two forks or a stand mixer. Add the shredded chicken to the ramekins, followed by the tomato and the cheese.

4. To finish, air-fry for 18 minutes or until it is done. Bon appétit!

298. Dinner Turkey Sandwiches

Servings: 4
Cooking Time: 4 Hours 30 Minutes
Ingredients:

- 1/2 pound turkey breast
- 1 teaspoon garlic powder
- 7 ounces condensed cream of onion soup
- 1/3 teaspoon ground allspice
- BBQ sauce, to savor

Directions:

1. Simply dump the cream of onion soup and turkey breast into your crock-pot. Cook on HIGH heat setting for 3 hours.
2. Then, shred the meat and transfer to a lightly greased baking dish.
3. Pour in your favorite BBQ sauce. Sprinkle with ground allspice and garlic powder. Air-fry an additional 28 minutes.
4. To finish, assemble the sandwiches; add toppings such as pickled or fresh salad, mustard, etc.

299. Spicy Eggs With Sausage And Swiss Cheese

Servings: 6
Cooking Time: 25 Minutes
Ingredients:

- 1 teaspoon lard
- 1/2 pound turkey sausage
- 6 eggs
- 1 scallion, chopped
- 1 garlic clove, minced
- 1 bell pepper, seeded and chopped
- 1 chili pepper, seeded and chopped
- Sea salt and ground black pepper, to taste
- 1/2 cup Swiss cheese, shredded

Directions:

1. Start by preheating your Air Fryer to 330 degrees F. Now, spritz 4 silicone molds with cooking spray.
2. Melt the lard in a saucepan over medium-high heat. Now, cook the sausage for 5 minutes or until no longer pink.
3. Coarsely chop the sausage; add the eggs, scallions, garlic, peppers, salt, and black pepper. Divide the egg mixture between the silicone molds. Top with the shredded cheese.
4. Bake in the preheated Air Fryer at 340 degrees F for 15 minutes, checking halfway through the cooking time to ensure even cooking. Enjoy!

300.Super Easy Sage And Lime Wings

Servings: 4
Cooking Time: 30 Minutes + Marinating Time
Ingredients:

- 1 teaspoon onion powder
- 1/3 cup fresh lime juice
- 1/2 tablespoon corn flour
- 1/2 heaping tablespoon fresh chopped parsley
- 1/3 teaspoon mustard powder
- 1/2 pound turkey wings, cut into smaller pieces
- 2 heaping tablespoons fresh chopped sage
- 1/2 teaspoon garlic powder
- 1/2 teaspoon seasoned salt
- 1 teaspoon freshly cracked black or white peppercorns

Directions:

1. Simply dump all of the above ingredients into a mixing dish; cover and let it marinate for about 1 hours in your refrigerator.
2. Air-fry turkey wings for 28 minutes at 355 degrees F. Bon appétit!

CPSIA information can be obtained
at www.ICGtesting.com
Printed in the USA
LVHW060824140121
676409LV00039B/394

9 781801 244800